HAND Acupuncture

CLINICAL TREATMENT

手临床疗法

Sumiko Knudsen

Ph.D
Practitioner. DK

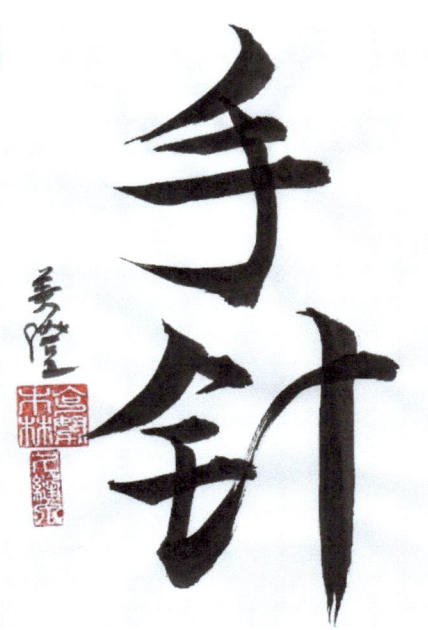

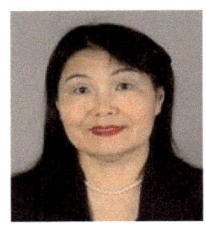

Sumiko Knudsen was born in Japan, and she has lived in USA, UK and Denmark for many years. She graduated at Nordic College of Chinese Acupuncture in Denmark, and then she went on and studied at Beijing University of TCM in China. After that she studied and graduated at Nanjing University of TCM in China. and she earned Ph.D. She is a private practitioner in Denmark.

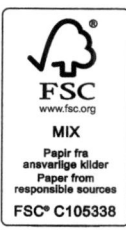

Forlag: BoD – Books on Demand, Hellerup, Danmark
Tryk: BoD – Books on Demand, Norderstedt, Tyskland

ISBN: 9788743045731

CONTENTS

Chrapter 3. Treatment of common diseases

I. Internal Medicine..79

INTRODUCTION

Hand Acupuncture therapy for the treatment of diseases is a therapeutic method applying different types of stimulation at various specific parts of the hand to promote circulation of Qi and Blood through meridians.

The specific parts of hand are classified as the regular points, extra points, and special points of the hand.

Since old days, we would automatically rub and press our hands on painful areas for promoting Qi and Blood circulation and to relieve, resolve swelling for correcting functional imbalances.

The hand is just like a window revealing some information of diseases.
The nails colour and shape condition have great value for treating instruction.

The hand can be used to diagnose and treat diseases as the hand is closely connected with other parts of the body in a common internal environment.

Hand therapy is safe, reliable, and easy to perform for both early diagnosis and treatment. Hand therapy is non-medicinal nature.

Therefore, it has attracted the attention of more people in the world.

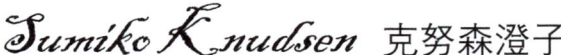 克努森澄子

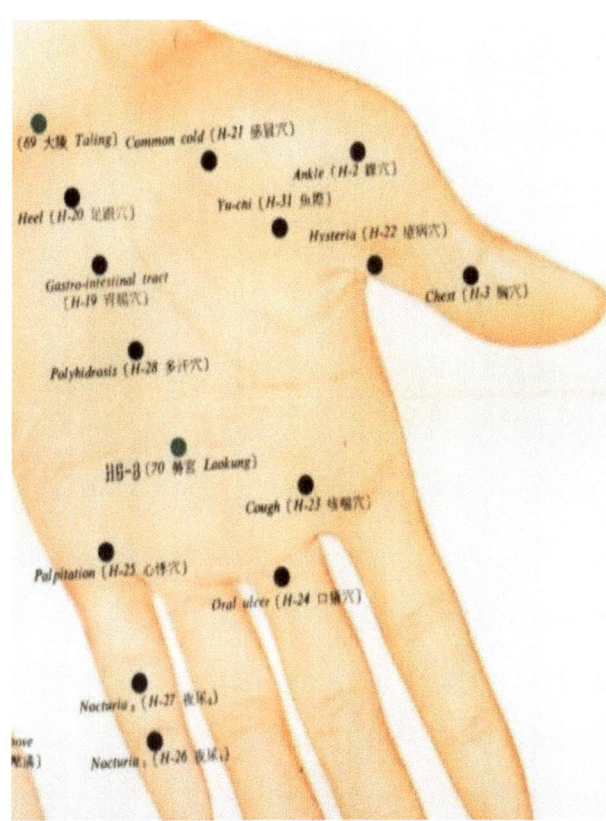

Acu points for hand therapy

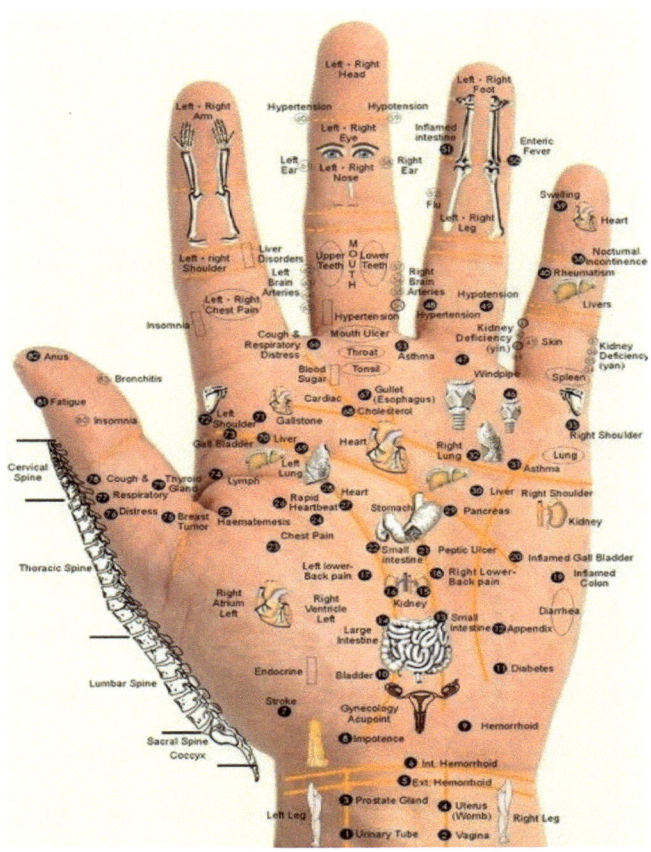

Hand pressure points acupressure massage therapy

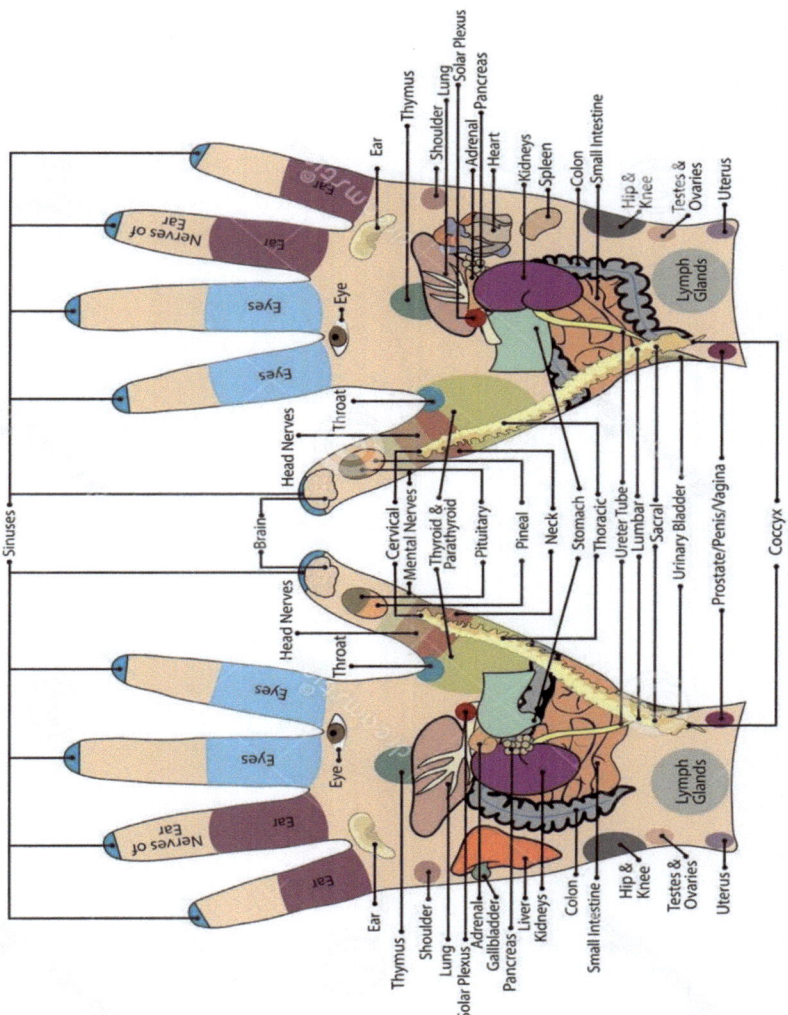

Chart of the hand reflective zones: Left and right dorsum of hand

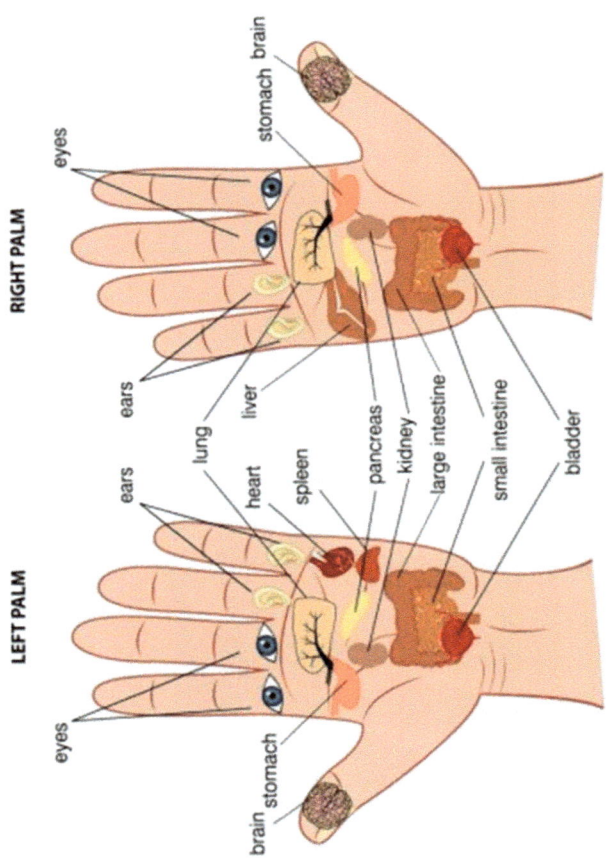

Acu pressure Zones: Left and right palm

Charpter 1. Common Acupuncture points for Hand Therapy

Acupuncture points for hand therapy include the regular and extra points on the hand. Acupuncture points on the forearm are also used in hand therapy.

I. The Lung Channel of Hand Taiyin
手太阴肺经经穴

1. LU-5 (Chize 尺泽)

- **He Sea point.**

- **Location**
  On the transverse cubital crease, in the depression at the radial side of the tendon of biceps brachii.

- **Function**
  To suppress adverse ascent of lung qi, tone lung yin, moisten the lung.

- **Indications**

Cough, Asthma, Dyspnea, Hemoptysis, fullness of the chest, afternoon fever, sore throat, spasmodic pain of the elbow and arm.

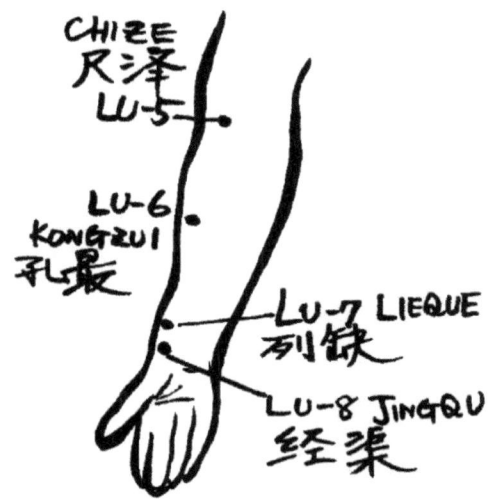

2. LU-6 (Kongzui 孔最)

- **Xi-Cleft point.**

- **Location**
  On the medial border of the radius, along the line connection LU-5, 5 cun below. 7 cun above the LU-9.)

- **Function**
  To suppress adverse ascent of lung qi, clear blood heat, stop bleeding.

- **Indications**
  Hemoptysis, cough, dyspnea, sore throat, hemorrhoids, aphonia, pain of the arm and elbow, headache.

3. LU-7 (Lieque 列缺)

- **Luo-Connecting point.**

- **Location**
  On the radial aspect of the forearm 1.5 cun above the transverse crease of the wrist between two tendons.

  When the index fingers and thumbs of both hands are crossed with the other hand, LU-7 is right under the tip of the index finger.

- **Function**
  To expel pathogen from lungs, adjust Ren.

- **Indications**
  Cough, asthma, migraine, hemoptysis, sore throat, stiff neck, toothache, feverish urination, pain in the penis and feverish sensation in the palms.

4. LU-8 (Jingqu 经渠)

- **Location**
  1 cun above the transverse crease of the wrist, in the depression on the lateral side of the radial artery.

- **Function**
  To control cough and asthma, breath.

- **Indications**
  Cough, asthma, sore throat, pain in the chest, pain in the wrist.

5. LU-9 (Taiyuan 太渊)

- **Yuan-Primary point.**

- **Location**
  At the radial end of transvers crease of the wrist, in the depression on the radial side of the radial artery.

- **Function**
  To control cough and resolve phlegm, improve body resistance, expel pathogens.

- **Indications**
  Cough, asthma, sore throat, palpitation, pain in the chest, wrist, arm.

6. LU-10 (Yuji 鱼际)

- **Location**
  At the radial aspect of the midpoint of the first metacarpal bone, on the junction of the red and white skin.

- **Function**
  To clear heat in lungs, relieve stagnation in throat, and clear heat in blood.

- **Indications**

Cough, hemoptysis, sore throat, aphonia, loss of voice, feverish sensation in the palms.

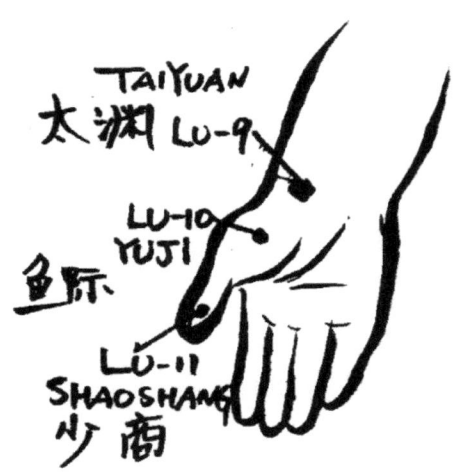

7. LU-11 (Shaoshang 少商)

- **Jing-Well point.**

- **Location**
  On the radial side of the thumb, 0.1 cun from the corner of the nail.

- **Function**
  To clear heat, open sense organ orifices, restore yang, revive critical patients, relieve stagnation in throat and control convulsion.

- **Indications**
  Cough, asthma, sore throat, epistaxis, abdominal fullness, mania, pain of the thumb.

II. The Large Intestine Channel of Hand-Yangming 手阳明大肠经经穴

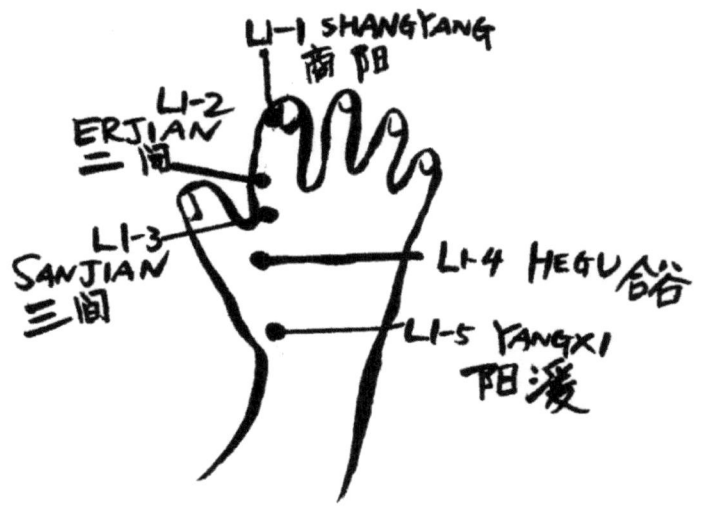

1. LI-1 (Shangyang 商阳)

- **Jing-Well point.**

- **Location**
  On the radial side of the index finger, 0.1 cun beside the corner of the nail.

- **Function**
  To clear heat, resolve swelling, open sense organ orifices, refresh the mind.

- **Indications**
  Apoplexy, coma, toothache, deafness, numbness of fingers, high fever.

2. LI-2 (Erjian 二间)

- **Location**
  On the radial side of the index finger, in the depression distal to the second metacarpal-phalangeal joint. Point locates slightly flexed.

- **Function**
  To clear heat and resolve swelling.

- **Indications**
  Toothache, sore throat, blurring of vision, facial paralysis, numbness of fingers.

3. LI-3 (Sanjian 三间)

- **Location**
  On the radial side of the index finger, in the depression proximal to the second metacarpal-phalangeal joint.

- **Function**
  To clear heat, resolve swelling, stop diarrhea.

- **Indications**
  Toothache, sore throat, epistaxis, swelling and pain of the dorsum of hand, numbness of fingers.

4. LI-4 (Hegu 合谷)

- **Yuan-Primary point.**

- **Location**
  On the dorsum of the hand between the first and second metacarpal bones, locate the point to stretch both thumbs and index finger of the left hand, place the transvers crease of the interphalangeal joint of the right thumb on the margin of the web between the left hand. The point is where the tip of the thumb touches.

- **Function**
  To clear heat, treat exterior syndrome, improve vision and hearing.

- **Indications**
  Swelling, redness and pain of eyes, headache, facial paralysis, epistaxis, sore throat, deafness, toothache, swelling of the face, common cold, cough, paralysis and spasm of fingers, infantile convulsion, irregular menstruation, delayed labour, obstruction syndrome in apoplexy, weakness and motor impairment.

5. LI-5 (Yangxi 阳溪)

- **Location**
  On the radial side of the wrist, when the thumb is tilted upward, it is the depression between the tendons of extensor pollicis longus and brevis.

- **Function**
  To clear heat, tranquilize the mind, improve vision, remove stagnation of the throat.

- **Indications**
  Headache, tinnitus, deafness, mania, epilepsy, spasmodic pain in the wrist, toothache, redness, pain, and swelling in the eyes.

6. LI-6 (Pianli 偏历)

- **Luo-Connecting point.**

- **Location**
  On the radial side of dorsal surface of the forearm, 3 cun proximal to the wrist crease.

- **Function**
  To improve vision and hearing.

- **Indications**
  Tinnitus, deafness, redness of the eye, spasmodic pain in the arm and hand, epistaxis, facial paralysis, sore throat, edema.

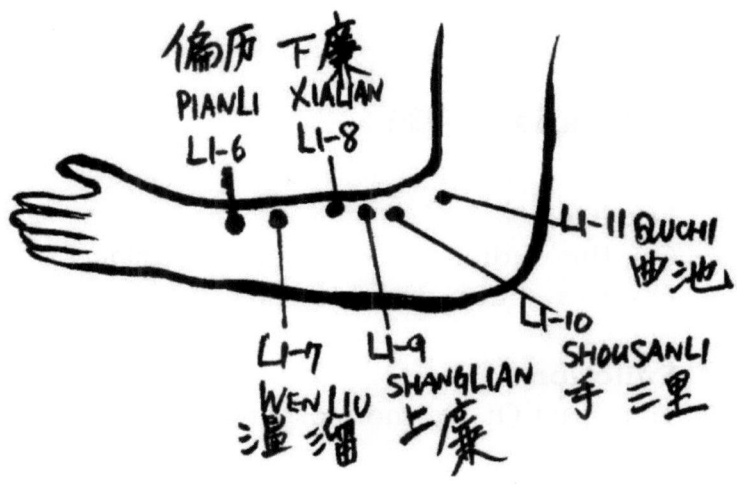

7. LI-7 (Wenliu 温溜)

- **Xi-Cleft point.**

- **Location**
  On the radial side of dorsal surface of the forearm, 5 cun proximal to the wrist crease.

- **Indications**

Headache, epistaxis, sore throat, abdominal pain, pain in the shoulder and arm.

8. LI-8 (Xialian 下廉)

- **Location**
  On the radial side of dorsal surface of the forearm, 4 cun distal to the cubital crease.

- **Function**
  To adjust Qi. Promote organs.

- **Indications**
  Abdominal pain, pain in the elbow and arm, motor impairment of the upper limbs.

9. LI-9 Shanglian (Shanglian 上廉)

- **Location**
  On the radial side of dorsal surface of the forearm, 3 cun distal to the cubital crease.

- **Function**
  To adjust Qi. Promote organs.

- **Indications**
  Motor impairment of the upper limbs, numbness of the hand and arm, pain in shoulder and arm, abdominal pain.

10. LI-10 (Shousanli 手三里)

- **Location**
  On the radial side of dorsal surface of the forearm, 2 cun distal to the cubital crease.

- **Function**
  To clear heat, improve vision, adjust Qi, promote organs.

- **Indications**
  Toothache, swelling of the cheek, abdominal pain, borborygmus, diarrhea, paralysis of the upper limbs, pain in the shoulder and back.

11. LI-11 (Quchi 曲池)

- **He-Sea point.**

- **Location**
  In the depression at the lateral end of the transverse cubital crease.

- **Function**
  To expel wind pathogen, control itching, clear heat, resolve swelling.

- **Indications**
  Toothache, redness and pain of eyes, sore throat, abdominal pain, diarrhea, paralysis of the upper limbs, spasmodic pain of the elbow and arm, febrile diseases, hypertension, urticaria.

III. The Heart Channel of Hand-Taiyang
手阴心经经穴

1. HT-3 (Shaohai 少海)

- **He-Sea point of the Heart channel.**

- **Location**
  When the elbow is flexed, at the midpoint of the line jointing the medial end of the transverse cubital crease.

- **Function**
  To tranquilize the mind.

- **Indications**
  Cardiac pain, mania, epilepsy, numbness of arm and hand, pain in the axilla, tremor of hand, scrofula, headache, toothache.

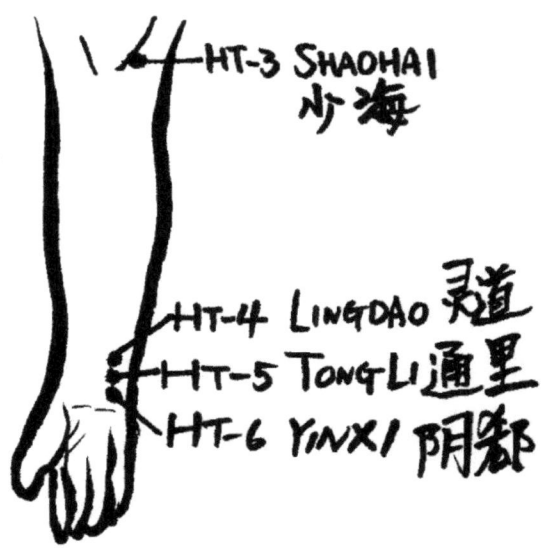

2. HT-4 (Lingdao 灵道)

- **Location**
  On the palm side of the forearm, 1.5 cun above
  the transverse crease of the wrist.

- **Function**
  To regulate Qi.
- **Indications**

Angina pectoris, palpitation, spasmodic pain of the elbow and arm, aphasia, sorrow and fright.

3. HT-5 (Tongli 通里)

- **Luo-Connecting point of the Heart channel.**

- **Location**
  On the palm side of the forearm, 1 cun above the transverse crease of the wrist.

- **Function**
  To tranquilize the mind, tone Yin, clear heart heat.

- **Indications**
  Palpitation, dizziness, sudden loss of voice, aphasia due to stiff tongue, pain in the wrist and arm.

4. HT-6 (Yinxi 阴郄)

- **Xi-Cleft point of the Heart channel.**

- **Location**
  On the palmer side of the forearm, 0.5 cun above the transverse crease of the wrist.

- **Function**
  To tranquilize the mind, clear heat in the blood.

- **Indications**
  Angina pectoris, palpitation, epistaxis, sudden loss of voice, epistaxis, blurring of vision.

5. HT-7 (Shenmen 神门)

- **Yuan-Source of the Heart channel.**
- **Location**
  At the ulnar end of the transverse crease of the wrist, on the radial side of flexor carpi ulnar, in the depression at the proximal border of the pisiform bone.

- **Function**
  To improve the body's resistance, expel pathogens, tranquilize the mind.

- **Indications**
Angina pectoris, Insomnia, palpitation, mania, epilepsy, hypochondriac pain, wrist pain, finger numbness, dementia.

6. HT-8 (Shaofu 少府)

- **Location**
On the palm, in the depression between the fourth and fifth metacarpal bones.
When a fist is made, the point is on where the tip of the little finger rests.

- **Function**
To clear heat of the heart, tranquilize the mind.

- **Indications**
Palpitation, chest pain, dysuria, enuresis, spasmodic pain of the little finger, pruritus of the external genitalia.

7. HT-9 (Shaochong 少冲)

- **Jing-Well point**

- **Location**
  On the radial side of the little finger, 0.1 cun beside the corner of the nail.

- **Function**
  To clear heat, control convulsions, tranquilize the mind.

- **Indications**
  Palpitation, angina pectoris, mania, loss of consciousness, febrile disease, hypochondriac pain.

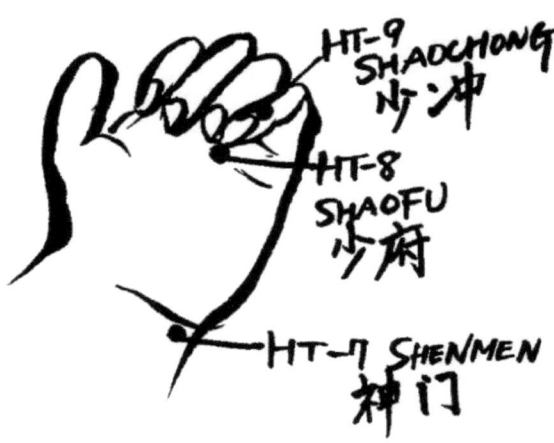

IV. The Small Intestine Channel of Hand-Taiyang 手太阳小肠经经穴

1. SI-1 (Shaoze 少泽)

- **Jing-Well point.**

- **Location**
  On the ulnar side of the little finger, 0.1 cun from the corner of the nail.

- **Function**
  To increase body fluid, promote discharge of milk, clear heat, facilitate discharge through orifices.

- **Indications**
  Apoplexy, loss of consciousness, cataract, tinnitus, deafness, sore throat, breast abscess, headache, febrile diseases.

2. SI-2 (Qiangu 前谷)

- **Location**

When a loose fist is made, the point on the ulnar end of the crease, side of the 5th metacarpophalangeal joint.

- **Function**
  To disperse Liver Qi, clear Heart heat, improve vision and hearing.

- **Indications**
  Headache, numbness of the fingers, tinnitus, deafness.

3. SI-3 (Houxi 后溪)

- **Location**
  When a loose fist is made, the point on the ulnar side of the hand, at the end of the transverse crease proximal to the fifth metacarpophalangeal joint.

- **Function**
  To clear Heart heat, relieve depression, control malaria with fever.

- **Indications**

Tinnitus, deafness, sore throat, mania, epilepsy, stiff neck, numbness of the fingers, pain in the shoulder and elbow, febrile diseases.

4. SI-4 (Wangu 腕骨)

- **Yuan-Source point of the Small Intestine Channel.**

- **Location**
  On the ulnar side of the hand, in the depression between the base of the fifth metacarpal bone and the triquetral bone.

- **Function**
  To increase body fluids, relieve thirst, promote the discharge of bile, reduce jaundice.

- **Indications**
  Tinnitus, deafness, numbness of fingers, febrile disease, jaundice, cataract, pain and stiffness of neck.

5. SI-5 (Yanggu 阳谷)

- **Location**
  At the ulnar side of the wrist, in the depression between styloid process of the ulna and the triquetral bone.

- **Function**
  To clear Heart heat, tranquilize the mind, improve vision and hearing.

- **Indications**
  Headache, tinnitus, deafness, mania, epilepsy, swelling and pain of the eyes, febrile disease,

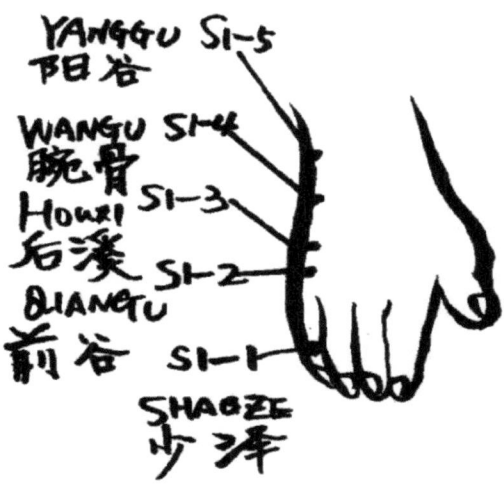

pain of the hand and wrist, swelling of the neck.

6. SI-6 (Yanglao 养老)

- **Xi-Cleft point of the Small Intestine channel.**

- **Location**
  With the palm facing downward, put a fingertip on the highest spot of the head of ulna, in a depression under the finger, on the radial side of the styloid process of the ulna.

- **Function**
  To increase body fluids for nourishing muscles, clear head, improve vision.

- **Indications**
  Blurred vision, pain in the shoulder, back, elbow and arm.

7. SI-7 (Zhizheng 支正)

- **Luo-connecting point of the Small Intestine channel.**

- **Location**
  On the line connecting SI-6 (Yanglao 养老) and SI-8(Xiaohai 小海), 5 cun proximal to the dorsal crease of the wrist.

- **Function**
  To disperse Liver Qi, tranquilize the mind, clear heat, treat exterior syndromes.

- **Indications**
  Headache, dizziness, depressive psychosis, mania, febrile diseases, pain in the elbow, arm and fingers.

8. SI-8 (Xiaohai 小海)

- **He-Sea point of the Small Intestine channel.**

- **Location**
  When the elbow is flexed, in the depression between the olecranon of the ulna and the tip of the medial epicondyle of the humerus.

- **Function**
  To disperse Liver Qi, tranquilize the mind, clear heat, resolve swelling.

- **Indications**
  Headache, dizziness, tinnitus, deafness, epilepsy, pain in the shoulder, arm and elbow.

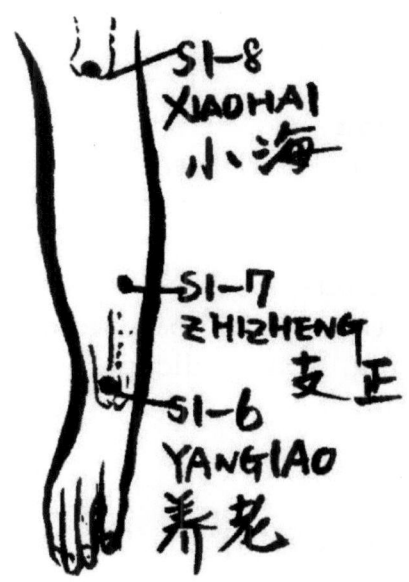

V. The Pericardium channel of Hand Jueyin 手蕨阴心包经经穴

1. P-3 (Quze 曲泽)

- **He-Sea point of the Pericardium channel.**

- **Location**
  At the midpoint of the transverse cubital crease, at the ulnar side of the tendon of biceps brachii.

- **Function**
  To clear Heart heat, control pain, adjust suppress adverse ascent Qi.

- **Indications**
  Angina pectoris, palpitation, stomachache, vomiting, spasmodic pain of the elbow and forearm.

2. P-4 (Ximen 郄门)

- **Location**

On the palmar side of the forearm, 5 cun above the transverse crease of the wrist, on the line connecting P-3 (Quze 曲泽) and P-7 (Daling 大陵), between the tendons of palmaris longus and flexor carpi radialis.

- **Function**
  To clear Heart heat, control cough, clear blood heat, stop bleeding.

- **Indications**
  Angina pectoris, palpitation, hemoptysis, chest pain, epistaxis, epilepsy.

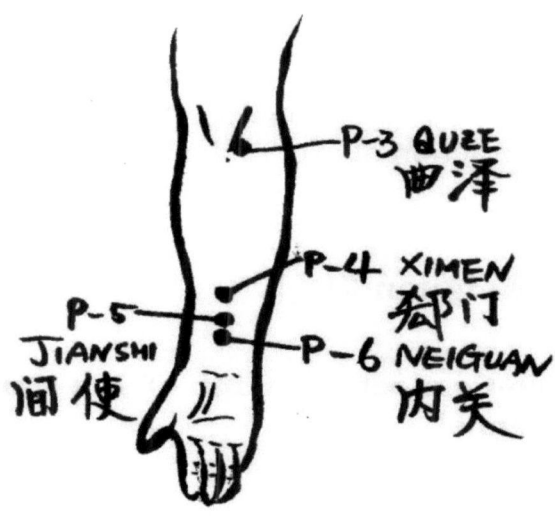

3. P-5 (Jianshi 间使)

- **Location**
  On the palmar side of the forearm, 3 cun above the transverse crease of the wrist, on the line connecting P-3 (Quze 曲泽) and P-7 (Daling 大陵), between the tendons of palmaris longus and flexor carpi radialis.

- **Function**
  To expand chest, relieve depression, tranquilize the mind, suppress adverse ascent of Qi.

- **Indications**
  Angina pectoris, palpitation, stomachache, vomiting, mania, malaria, epilepsy, contraction of arm and elbow.

4. P-6 (Neiguan 内关)

- **Luo-Connecting point of the Pericardium channel.**

- **Location**

On the palmar side of the forearm, 2 cun above the transverse crease of the wrist, on the line connecting P-3 (Quze 曲泽) and P-7 (Daling 大陵), between the tendons of palmaris longus and flexor carpi radialis.

- **Function**
  To tranquilize the mind, control pain, disperse Liver Qi, regulate Spleen and Stomach.

- **Indications**
  Angina pectoris, palpitation, stomachache, vomiting, nausea, epilepsy, insomnia, mental disorders, spasmodic pain elbow and arm, migraine, febrile disease.

5. P-7 (Daling 大陵)

- **Yuan-Source of the Pericardium channel.**
- **Location**
  On the palmar side of the forearm, at the midpoint of the transverse crease of the wrist, between the tendons of palmaris longus and flexor carpi radialis.

- **Function**
  To tranquilize the mind, expand chest, regulate Stomach.

- **Indications**
  Angina pectoris, palpitation, stomachache, mania, insomnia, pain in the hypochondriac region, vomiting.

6. P-8 (Laogong 劳宫)

- **Location**
  On the palm, between the second and third metacarpal bones. When the fist is made, the point is below the tip of the middle finger.

- **Function**
  To clear heat, tranquilize the mind, reduce swelling, stop itching.

- **Indications**
  Angina pectoris, palpitation, vomiting, epilepsy, mania, coma due to apoplexy.

7. P-9 (Zhongchong 中冲)

- **Jing-Well point.**

- **Location**
  At the center of the tip of the middle finger.

- **Function**
  To open sense organ orifices, restore consciousness, clear Heart heat.

- **Indications**
  Angina pectoris, palpitation, apoplexy, sunstroke, stiffness and swelling of the tongue, febrile disease.

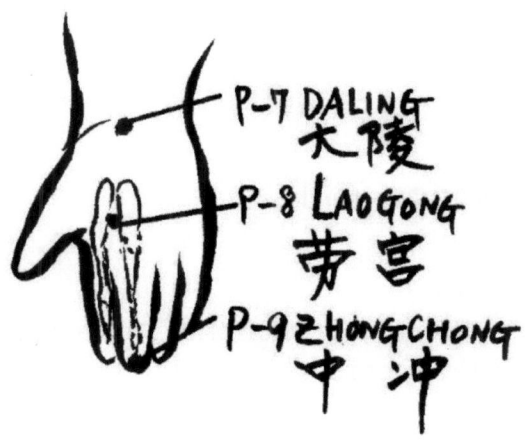

VI. The Sanjiao Channel of Hand Shaoyang
手少阳三焦经经穴

1. SJ-1 (Guanchong 关冲)

- **Jing-Well point.**
- **Location**
  On the ulnar side of the ring finger, 0.1 cun beside the corner of the nail.

- **Function**
  To clear heat, treat exterior syndrome, clear Heart heat, improve hearing.

- **Indications**
  Apoplexy, headache, tinnitus, deafness, redness of the eyes.

2. SJ-2 (Yemen 液门)

- **Location**
  When the fist is clenched, between the ring and little fingers, proximal to the margin of the web.

- **Function**
  To clear Heart heat, improve hearing, regulate organ functions.

- **Indications**
  Headache, redness of the eyes, tinnitus, deafness, sore throat, numbness of fingers.

3. SJ-3 (Zhongzhu 中诸)

- **Location**
  On the dorsum of the hand between the fourth and fifth the metacarpal bones, in the depression proximal to the 4metacarpophalangeal joint, 1 cun posterior to SJ-2 (Yemen 液门).

- **Function**
  To clear heat, remove stagnation in throat, improve vision and hearing.

- **Indications**
  Headache, dizziness, tinnitus, deafness redness of the eyes, sore throat, pain in the elbow and arm, spasmodic pain of the fingers.

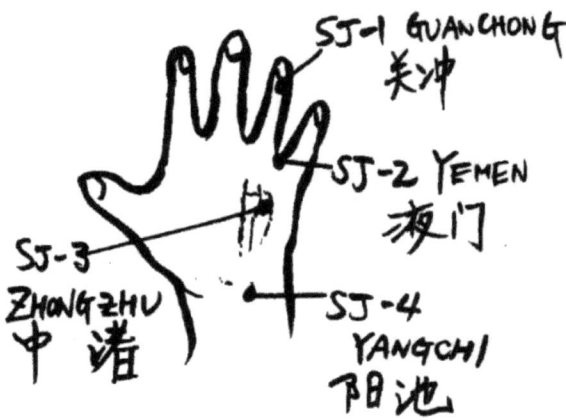

4. SJ-4 (Yangchi 阳池)

- **Yuan-Source point of the Sanjiao channel.**
- **Location**
  On the dorsum of the wrist, in the depression between the tendons of extensor digitorum communis and extensor digiti minimi.

- **Function**
  To remove stagnation in throat, improve hearing, regulate organ functions

- **Indications**

Tinnitus, deafness, sore throat, pain in the arm, and wrist, flaccidity and Bi syndrome of the upper limbs, diabetes.

5. SJ-5 (Waiguan 外关)

- **Luo-Connecting point of the Sanjiao channel.**

- **Location**
  On the dorsum of the forearm, on the line connecting SJ-4 (Yangchi 阳池) and olecranon, 2 cun proximal to the dorsal crease of the wrist, between the radius and the ulna.

- **Function**
  To treat exterior syndrome, clear heat, improve hearing and vision.

- **Indications**
  Deafness, tinnitus, migraine, pain in the cheek, headache, febrile disease, motor impairment of the elbow and arm.

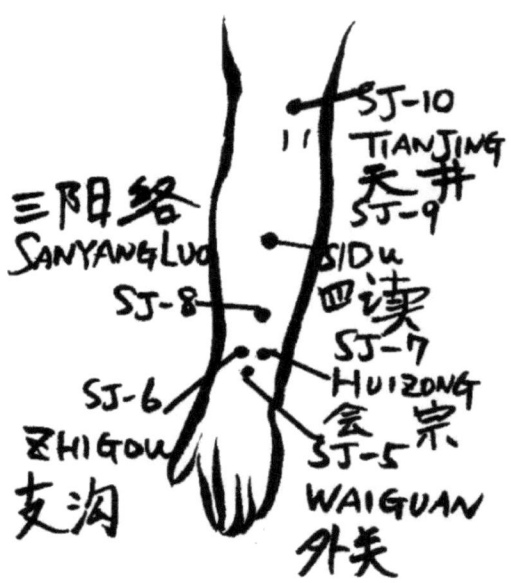

6. SJ-6 (Zhigou 支沟)

- **Location**
  On the dorsum of the forearm, on the line connecting SJ-4 (Yangchi 阳池) and olecranon, 3 cun proximal to the dorsal crease of the wrist, between the radius and the ulna.

- **Function**

To clear heat, improve hearing, suppress adverse ascent of Qi, moisten intestines.

- **Indications**
  Tinnitus, deafness, pain in the shoulder and back, sudden loss of voice, pain in the hypochondriac region, constipation, vomiting.

7. SJ-7 (Huizong 会宗)

- **Xi-Cleft point of the Sanjiao channel.**

- **Location**
  On the dorsum of the forearm, at the same level with SJ-6 (Zhigou 支沟), on the radial border of the ulna.

- **Function**
  To improve hearing, control convulsions.

- **Indications**
  Pain in the ear, deafness, pain in the upper limbs.

8. SJ-8 (Sanyangluo 三阳络)

- **Location**
  On the dorsum of the forearm, 4 cun above the transverse crease, between the ulna and the radius.

- **Function**
  To improve hearing, remove stagnation in throat.

- **Indications**
  Deafness, sudden loss of voice, pain in the upper limbs.

9. SJ-9 (Sidu 四读)

- **Location**
  On the dorsum of the forearm, 7 cun proximal to SJ-4 (Yangchi 阳池), in the depression between the radius and the ulna.

- **Function**
  To improve hearing, remove stagnation in throat.

- **Indications**
  Deafness, sudden loss of voice, pain in the upper limbs.

10. SJ-10 (Tianjing 天井)

- **He-Sea point of the Sanjiao channel.**

- **Location**
  With the elbow flexed, in the depression 1 cun proximal to the tip of the olecranon.

- **Function**
  To improve hearing, tranquilize the mind, adjust Qi, resolve phlegm.

- **Indications**
  Migraine, pain in the shoulder and arm, epilepsy, hypochondriac pain.

VII. Extra-ordinary Point 常用经外奇穴定位

1. EX-UE1 (Zhoujian 肘尖

- **Location**
  On the posterior side of the elbow, at the tip of the ulnar olecranon when the elbow is flexed.

- **Function**
  To resolve phlegm and swelling.

- **Indications**
  Scrofula

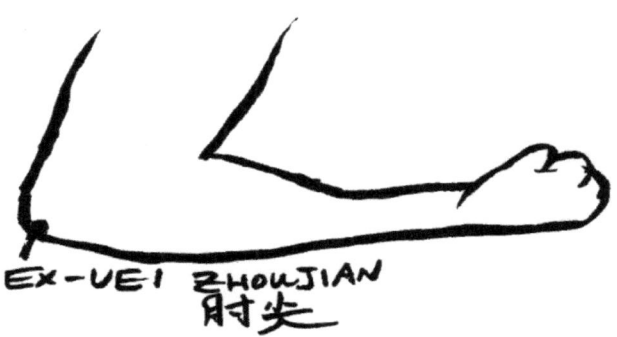

EX-UE1 ZHOUJIAN
肘尖

2. EX-UE2 (Erbai 二白)

- **Location**
  On the palmar side of forearm, a pair of points, 4 cun above the transverse crease of the wrist, on both sides of the tendon of m. flexor carpi radialis, two points on the hand.

- **Function**
  To replace prolapse of rectum, treat hemorrhoids.

- **Indications**
  Hemorrhoids, prolapse of the rectum.

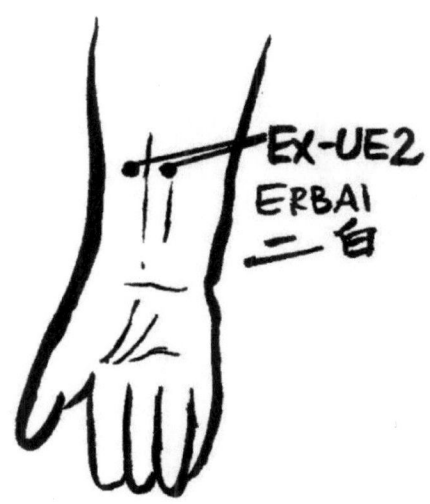

3. EX-UE4 (Zhongkui 中魁)

- **Location**
  On the dorsal side of the middle finger, at the center of the proximal interphalangeal joint.
- **Function**
  To suppress adverse ascent of Qi, regulate stomach.

- **Indications**
  Nausea, hiccup, vomiting.

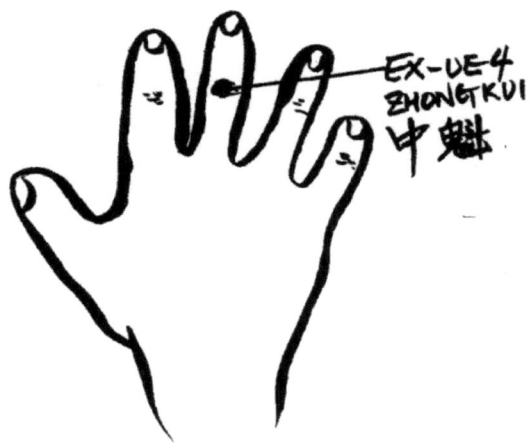

4. EX-UE5 (Dagukong 大骨空)

- **Location**
  On the dorsal side of the thumb, at the center of the interphalangeal joint.

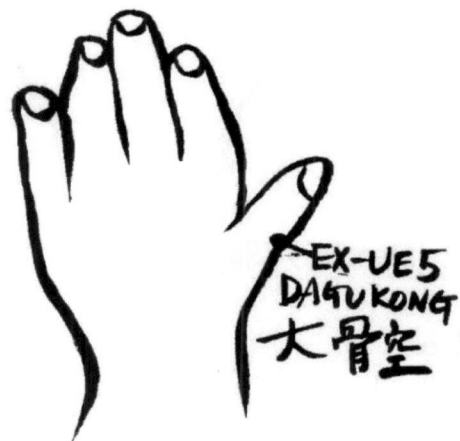

5. EX-UE6 (Xiaogukong 小骨空)

- Location
  On the dorsal side of the little finger, at the midpoint of the proximal interphalangeal joint.

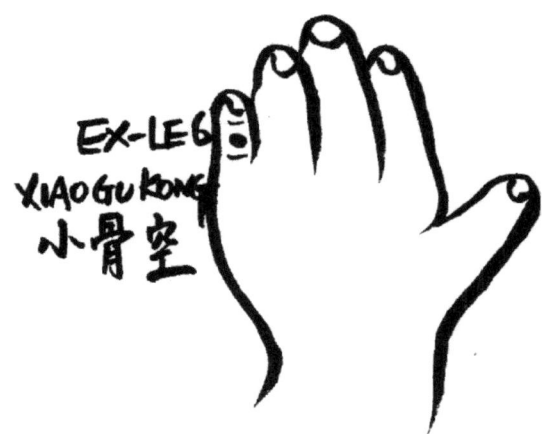

EX-LE6
XIAOGU KONG
小骨空

6. EX-UE9 (Baxie 八邪)

- **Location**
  When the hand is made into a fist, the points are located at the ends of the vertical skin crease of the webs between every two fingers.

- **Function**
  To clear heat, reduce swelling.

- **Indications**
  Spasm, numbness, of the fingers, swelling and pain of the dorsum of the hand.

7.EX-UE10 (Sifeng 四缝)

- **Location**

  On the palmar side of the hand, in the midpoint of the transverse crease of the proximal interphalangeal joint of the index, middle, ring and small fingers.

- **Function**

  To strengthen spleen, release stagnation of food.

- **Indications**

  Whooping cough, indigestion syndrome in children.

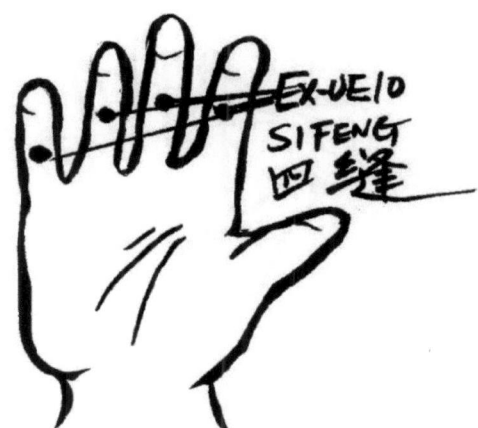

8. EX-UE11 (Shixuan 十宣)

- **Location**
  On the tips of the ten fingers, 0.1cun distal to the nails.

- **Function**
  To open sense organ orifices, restore consciousness, clear heat, control convulsions.

- **Indications**
  Numbness of fingertips, apoplexy, high fever, coma, tonsilitis, epilepsy.

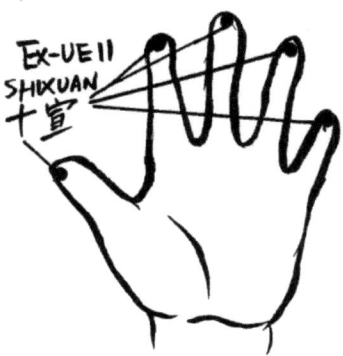

Charpter 2. Hand Therapy Methods

I. Hand Therapy Massage

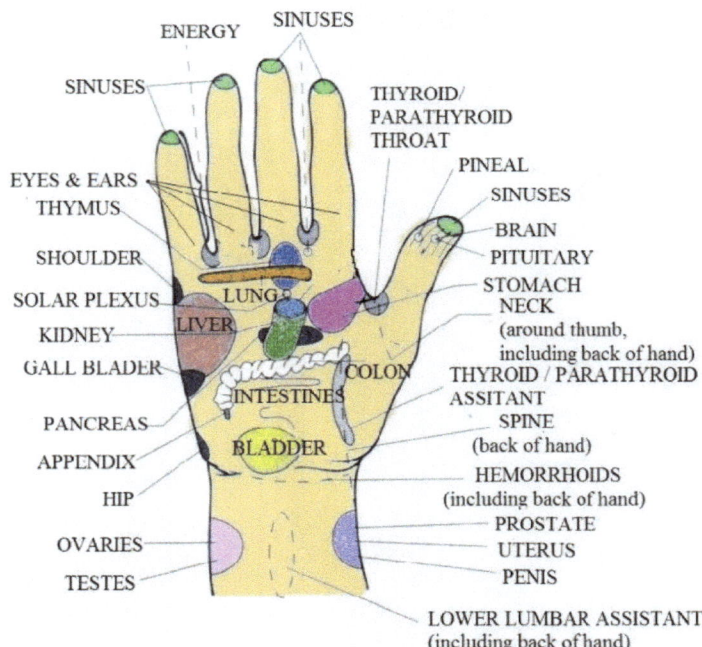

Acupressure points on the palm

In hand therapy massage, stimulation is applied by hand to the regular and extra acupoints, reflective points and reflective areas closely related to various internal organs and tissues in the body. The basic maneuvers of massage include pressing, digit pressing, kneading, pushing, pinching, twisting, rotating, pulling, rubbing, and grinding methods.

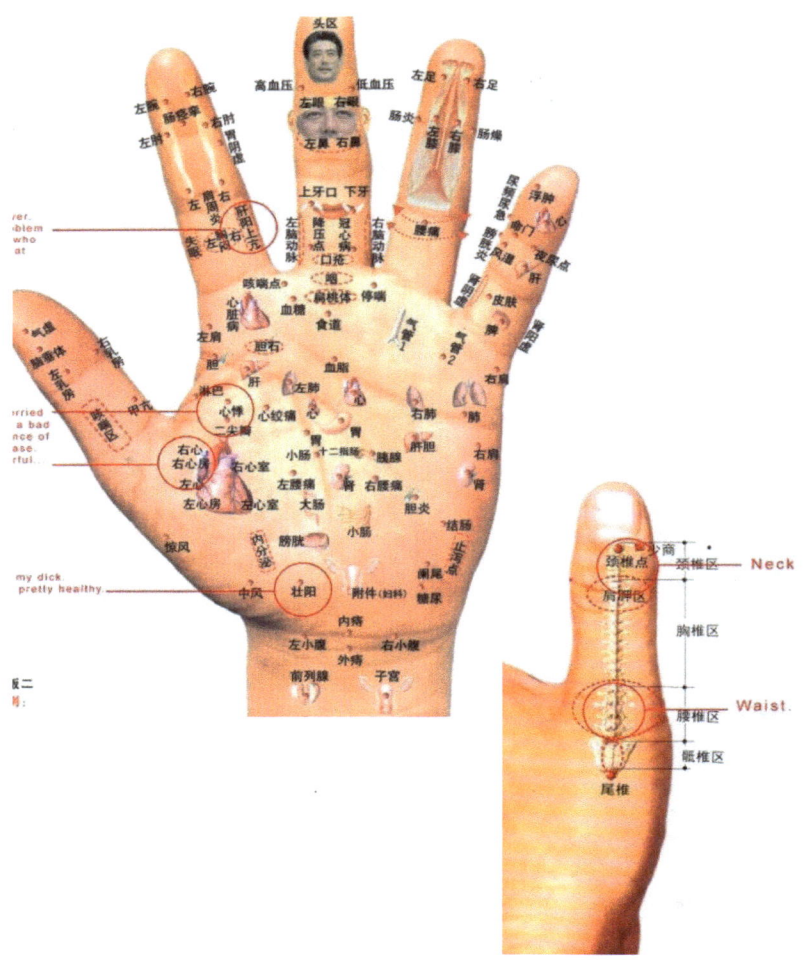

II. Hand Therapy Acupuncture

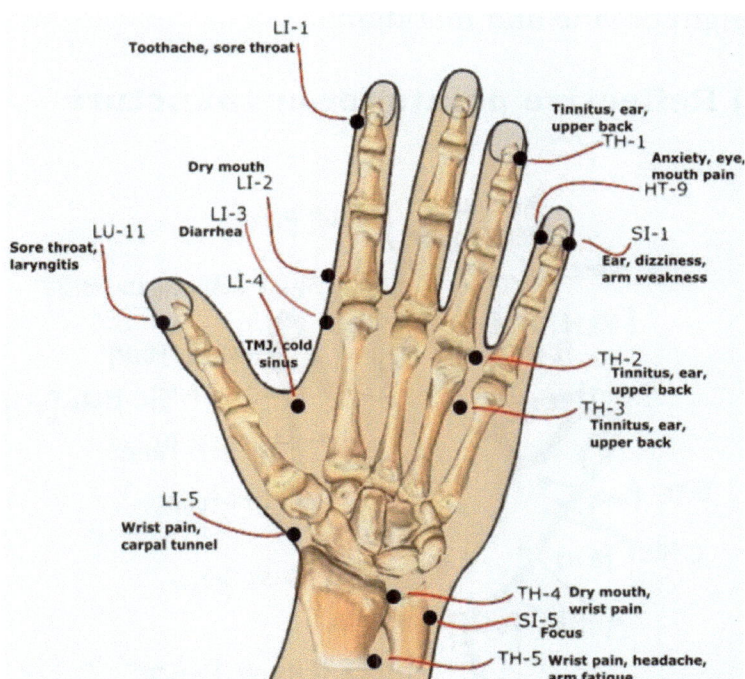

Acupuncture for hand therapy includes acupuncture at regular and extra points of the hand, acupuncture at reflective points of the hand and area, and acupuncture at special acupoints beside the second metacarpal bone.

1. Acupuncture at reflective points

This is a type of hand therapy to prevent and treat various diseases. The hands are closely related to Zangfu organs and meridians.

(1) Reflective points for acupuncture

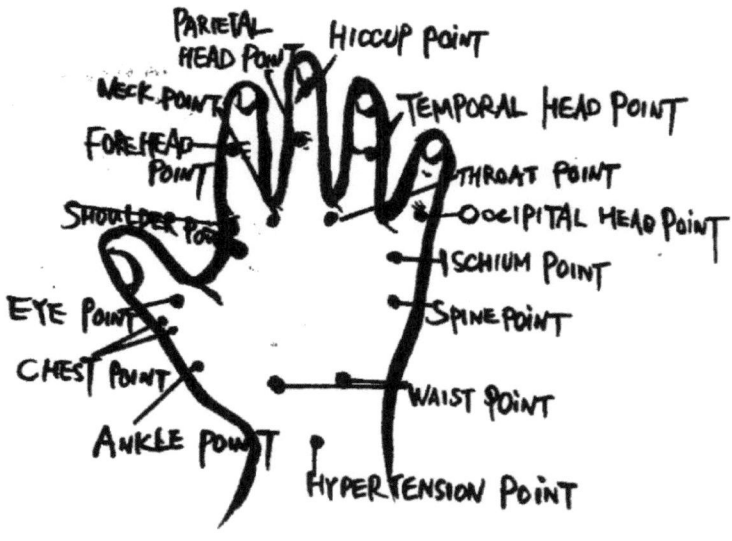

Reflective point of back of the hand

1) Waist point
- Location
  Five cm distal to dorsal crease of wrist, on the radial side of tendon of the second digital

extensor muscle and on the ulnar side of tendon of the fourth digital extensor muscle.

- Indications
  Lumbago and muscular sprain of waist.

2) Hypertension point
- Location
  At the midpoint of dorsal crease of wrist.

- Indications
  To reduce blood pressure.

3) Spine point
- Location
  On the ulnar side of metacarpophalangeal joint of little finger and on the dorsopalmar boundary of hand.

- Indications
  Lumbago, muscular sprain of waist, and tinnitus.

4) Ischium point
- Location

Between the fourth and fifth metacarpophalangeal joints and near the former joint.

- Indications
  Neuralgia, sciatica, and hip joint pain.

5) Throat point
  - Location
    Between the third and fourth metacarpophalangeal joints and near the former joint.

  - Indications
    Sore throat, toothache, and trigeminal neuralgia.

6) Neck point
  - Location
    Between the second and third metacarpophalangeal joints and near the former joint.

  - Indications
    Stiff neck and pain in neck and nape.

7) Shoulder point
- Location
  On the radial side of the second metacarpophalangeal joint and on the dorsopalmar boundary of hand.

- Indications
  Shoulder pain.

8) Eye point
- Location
  On the ulnar side of interphalangeal joint of thumb and on the dorsopalmar boundary of hand.

- Indications
  Eye diseases.

9) Forehead point
- Location
  On the radial side of proximal interphalangeal joint of index finger and on the dorsopalmar boundary of hand.

- Indications
  Frontal headache, diseases of stomach and intestines, and knee and ankle joint pain.

10) Parietal head point
- Location
On the radial side of proximal interphalangeal joint of middle finger and on the dorsopalmar boundary of hand.

- Indications
Parietal headache.

11) Temporal head point
- Location
On the ulnar side of proximal interphalangeal joint of ring finger and on the dorsopalmar boundary of hand.

- Indications
Migraine and chest and flank pain caused by diseases of the liver and gallbladder.

12) Occipital head point
- Location
On the ulnar side of proximal interphalangeal joint of little finger and on the dorsopalmar boundary of hand.

- Indications

Occipital headache and tonsillitis.

13) Hiccup point
- Location
  At the midpoint of dorsal crease of distal interphalangeal f middle finger.

- Indications
  Hiccups.

14) Heel point
- Location
  At the midpoint of a connecting line between stomach and intestine point and P-7 (Daling 大陵) point.

- Indications
  Heel pain.

(2) Reflective point of Palm side of hand

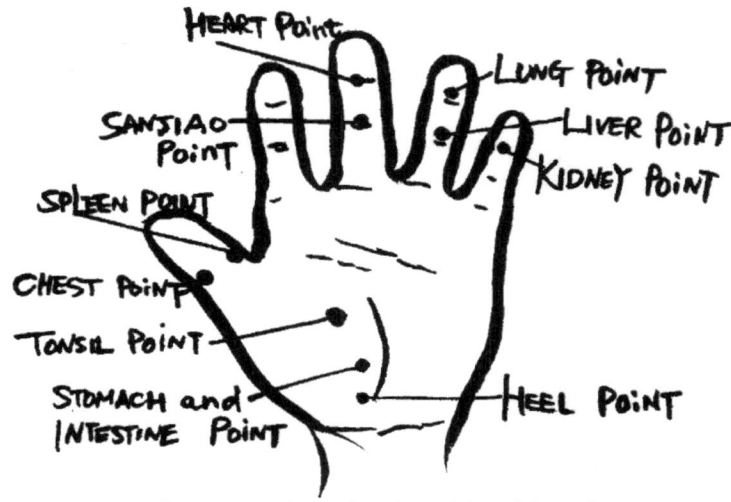

Reflective point of palm side of hand

1) Tonsil point
- Location
  On the palm and at the midpoint of ulnar border of the first metacarpal bone.

- Indications
  Tonsillitis and laryngitis.

2) Stomach and intestine point
- Location
  At the midpoint of a connecting line between P-8 (Laogong 劳宫) and P-7 (Daling 大陵) points.

- Indications
  Various diseases of the stomach and intestines.

3) Ankle point
  - Location
    On the radial side of metacarpophalangeal joint of thumb and on the dorsopalmar boundary of hand.

  - Indications
    Ankle joint pain.

4) Kidney (bed-wetting) point
  - Location
    On the palmar surface and at the midpoint of distal interphalangeal crease of little finger.

  - Indications
    Bed-wetting at night and frequent urination.

5) Spleen point
  - Location
    On the palmar surface and at the midpoint of interphalangeal crease of thumb.

  - Indications

Digestive system diseases.

6) Sanjiao point
- Location
  On the palmar surface and at the midpoint of proximal interphalangeal crease of middle finger.

- Indications
  Chest and abdomen diseases.

7) Heart point
- Location
  On the palmar surface and at the midpoint of distal interphalangeal crease of middle finger.

- Indications
  Cardiovascular diseases.

8) Liver point
- Location
  On the palmar surface and at the midpoint of proximal interphalangeal crease of ring finger.

- Indications
  Liver and Gallbladder diseases.

9) Lung point
- Location
  On the palmar surface and at the midpoint of distal interphalangeal crease of ring finger.

- Indications
  Respiratory system diseases.

10) Chest point
- Location
  On the radial side of interphalangeal joint of thumb and on the dorsopalmar boundary.

- Indications
  Chest pain, vomiting, and diarrhea.

11) Cough and Asthma point
- Location
  On the palmar surface and on the ulnar side of proximal interphalangeal joint of index finger.

- Indications
  Bronchitis and bronchial asthma.

Charpter 3. Treatment of common diseases

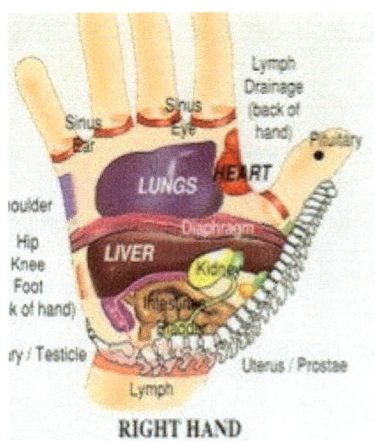

Massage zone: Right and Left palm

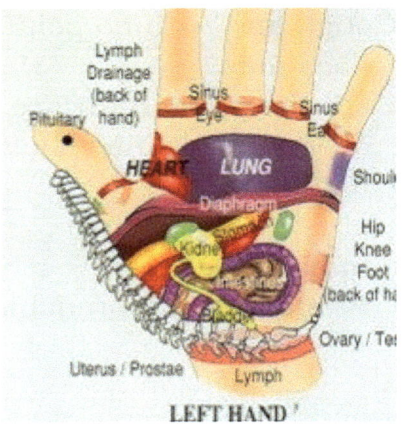

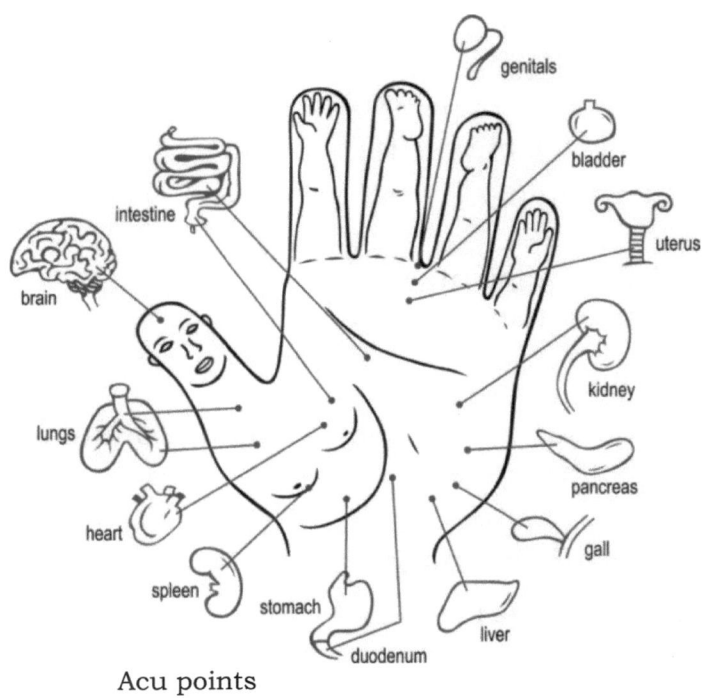

Acu points

I. Internal Medicine

1-1 Abdominal pain 腹痛 Futong

It is a common symptom with pain in the abdomen below the epigastric region and above the pubic symphysis. Acute pain in pancreatitis, gastric, intestinal colic, strangulated hernia, gastric, intestinal neurosis, and indigestion.

- Treatment
  Acupuncture point:
  LI-11 (Quchi 曲池), LI-4 (Hegu 合谷), P-6 (Neiguan 内关)

  Reflective point:
  Stomach and Intestine.

  Reflective area:
  Abdomen area in corresponding painful region of palmar reflective areas.

1-2 Abdominal mass 腹部肿块 Fubuzhongkuai

Abdominal mass, pain, distension, abdominal tumors, stomach dysfunction, intestinal obstruction, enlargement of the Liver and Spleen.

- Treatment
  Acupuncture point:
  LI-11 (Quchi 曲池), LI-10 (Shousanli 手三里), LI-4 (Hegu 合谷)

  Reflective point

Stomach and Intestine, Sanjiao

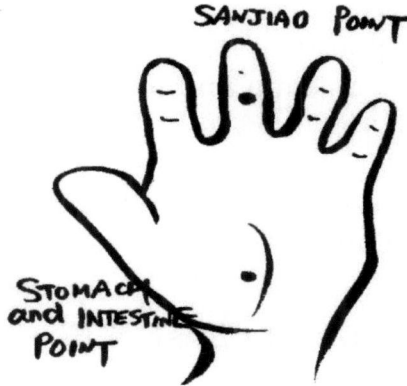

Stomach, Intestine, Sanjiao reflective point

1-3 Asthma 哮喘 **Xiaochuan**

It is characterized by paroxysmal attacks of gasping, difficulty breathing, and a whistling noise in the throat. This is caused by an accumulation of phlegm, constriction of the respiratory tract, and interference with pulmonary ventilation producing gasps and a whistling sound.

- Treatment
  Acupuncture point:

P-6 (Neiguan 内关), LU-5 (Chize 尺泽), LU-9 (Taiyuan 太渊)

Reflective points
Cough and asthma and lung.

Reflective area
Lung area of palmar reflective and radial reverse palmar reflective areas.

1-4 Bi-Syndrome of chest 胸痹 Xiongbizheng

This is characterized by distension and pain in the chest radiated to the back, and shortness of breath. Mild cases only feel fullness in the chest, while severe cases may suffer from heart pain radiated to the back and back pain radiated to the heart.

- Treatment
  Acupuncture point:
  P-6 (Neiguan 内关), P-5 (Jianshi 间使)
  Reflective points:
  Heart point and chest point.

  Massage:

Heart reflective point.
Heart area (thumb and middle finger): Palm side of hand.
HT-7 (Shenmen 神门), LU-11 (Shaoshang 少商), HT-9 (Shaochong 少冲)

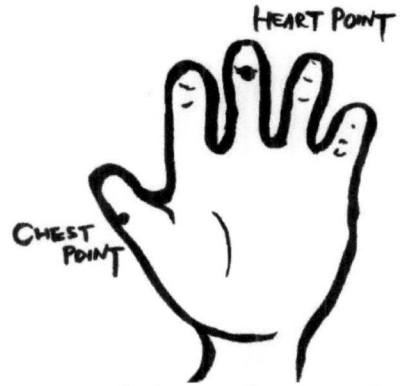

Heart and chest reflective point

1-5 Bi-Syndrome 痹症 Bizheng

This is characterized by numbness, heaviness, limited movement, swollen joints.

- Treatment
  Massage:
  Forehead reflective point.
  Joints of finger, wrist, palmar and dorsal interosseous spaces.

LI-4 (Hegu 合谷), LI-5 (Yangxi 阳溪), SJ-4 (Yangchi 阳池)

Reflective point:
Waist and Leg point, EX-UE8 (Wailaogong 外劳宫), forehead point.

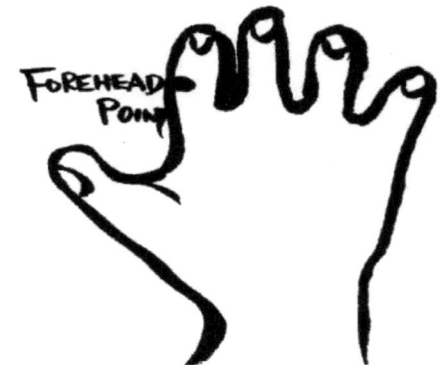

Forehead reflective point

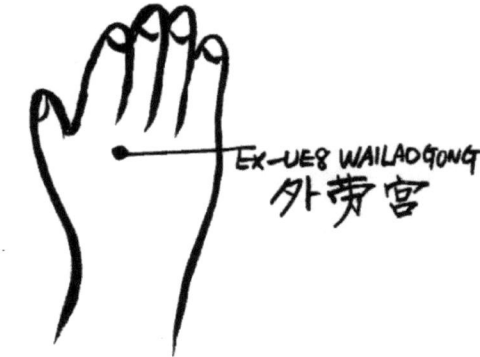

1-6 Common cold 普通感 **Putongganmao**

It is caused by an attack of external pathogens. The clinical symptoms include nasal obstruction, running nose, sneezing, cough, headache, chills, fever.

- Treatment
  Acupuncture point:
  LI-11 (Quchi 曲池), SJ-5 (Waiguan 外关), LI-4 (Hegu 合谷)

  Massage:
  Head reflective point.
  Lung area, nose and throat area, chest area.
  LI-4 (Hegu 合谷), LU-9 (Taiyuan 太渊)
  Reflective point:
  Lung point

1-7 Cough 咳嗽 **Kesou**

Coughing is symptom of respiratory system diseases. Coughing and spitting sputum are usually present at the same time.

- Treatment

Acupuncture point:
LU-7 (Lieque 列缺), LU-5 (Chize 尺泽)

Massage:
Lung reflective point.
Cough controlling point.
Nose and throat area, lung area and thenar prominence.
LU-9 (Taiyuan 太渊), LU-10 (Yuji 鱼际), HT-8 (Shaofu 少府)), LU-11 (Shaoshang 少商), LI-4 (Hegu 合谷), EX-UE10 (Sifeng 四缝)
Reflective point:
Lung point

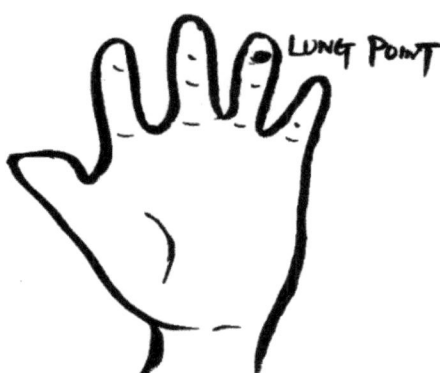

Lung reflective point

1-8 Constipation 便秘 Bianmi

This is characterized by hard stools difficult to pass, and prolonged intervals between bowel movements.

- Treatment
  Acupuncture point:
  SJ-6 (Zhigou 支沟), LI-4 (Hegu 合谷)

  Massage:
  On the side of palm, proximal ends of finger and web border between fingers.
  Intestine area, anus area, and digestive tract.
  LI-2 (Erjian 二间), LI-3 (Sanjian 三间), LI-4 (Hegu 合谷), central part of palm, proximal ends of finger and web border between fingers.

1-9 Diarrhea 泄泻 Xiexie

Loose or watery stool may be frequently passed due to diseases of the Spleen, Stomach, Large intestine, Small intestine.

- Treatment
  Acupuncture point:
  LI-11 (Quchi 曲池), LI-4 (Hegu 合谷), LI-10 (Shousanli 手三里)
  Massage:

Chest, stomach and intestine reflective point. Chest and abdomen area.
LI-3 (Sanjian 三间), EX-UE-5 (Dagukong 大骨空
*) * Diarrhea point

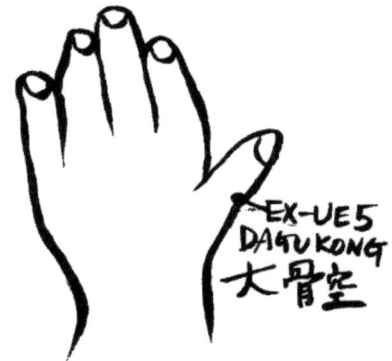

On the dorsal side of the thumb, at the center of the interphalangeal joint.

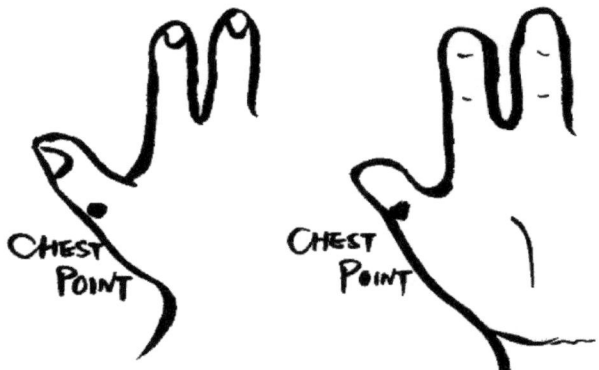

Chest reflective point of palm and dorsum
Stomach and Intestine reflective point

1-10 Dysentery 痢疾 **Liji**

It is with symptoms of abdominal pain, tenesmus and diarrhea with blood and pus in stool.

- Treatment
  Acupuncture point:

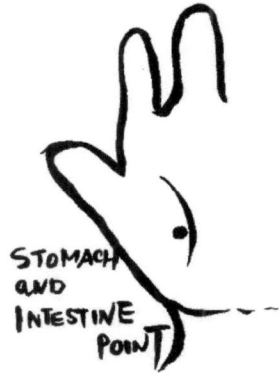

STOMACH and INTESTINE POINT

LI-11 (Quchi 曲池), LI-4 (Hegu 合谷)

Massage:
Stomach area, intestinal area, urinary bladder area, kidney area, dorsal interosseous spaces.
LI-3 (Sanjian 三间), EX-UE5 (Dagkong 大骨空*)

* Diarrhea point

1-11 Diabetes mellitus 糖尿病 **Tangniaobing**

The symptoms are excessive thirst, overeating, polyuria, sweet, turbid urine.

- Treatment
  Acupuncture point:
  SJ-4 (Yangchi 阳池), SI-7 (Zhizheng 支正), LU-10 (Yuji 鱼际)

  Massage:
  Throat, mouth, esophagus, stomach, and kidney area.
  LU-9 (Taiyuan 太渊), P-7 (Daling 大陵), SJ-4 (Yangchi 阳池)

1-12 Stomachache 腹痛 Futong

This is with pain of the epigastric area.

- Treatment
  Acupuncture point:
  P-6 (Neiguan 内关), LI-4 (Hegu 合谷)

  Massage:
  Stomach and Intestine reflective point.
  Midline of palm, intestine area, stomach area, spleen area.

P-7 (Daling 大陵)

Rubbing maneuver applied at central part of palm, pushing and pressing maneuvers along midline of palm.

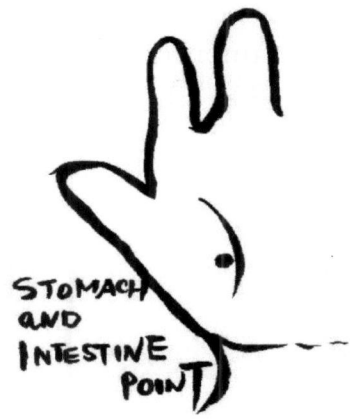

Stomach and Intestine reflective point

1-13 Epilepsy 癲癇 Dianxian

This is a paroxysmal attack of mental confusion, sudden collapse, loss of consciousness, forming at the mouth, upward staring of eyes and convulsion of limbs with noise cried from mouth.

- Treatment
  Acupuncture point:

P-6 (Neiguan 内关), LI-4 (Hegu 合谷), P-8 (Laogong 劳宫)

Massage:
Chest reflective point of palm and dorsum hand.HT-7 (Shenmen 神门), P-8 (Laogong 劳宫), LI-4 (Hegu 合谷), SI-3 (Houxi 后溪), SI-5 (Yanggu 阳谷), EX-UE11 (Shixuan 十宣) Chest

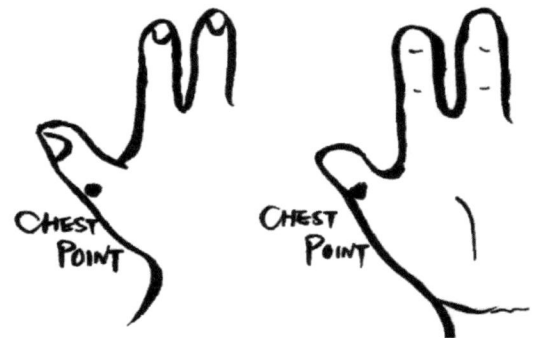

reflective point of palm and dorsum hand

1-14 Headache 头痛 Toutong

This is a common symptom that may occur alone or in conjunction with many acute and chronic diseases.

- Treatment
  Acupuncture point:

Frontal headache: LI-4 (Hegu 合谷)
Occipital headache: SI-3 (Houxi 后溪)
Temporal headache: SJ-3 (Zhongzhu 中诸)

Massage:
Head reflective point. (forehead, parietal head, temporal head and occipital head).
Brain area, kidney area.
LU-10 (Yuji 鱼际), LI-4 (Hegu 合谷), LI-5 (Yangxi 阳溪), SI-2 (Qiangu 前谷), SI-3 (Houxi 后溪), SJ-1 (Guanchong 关冲)

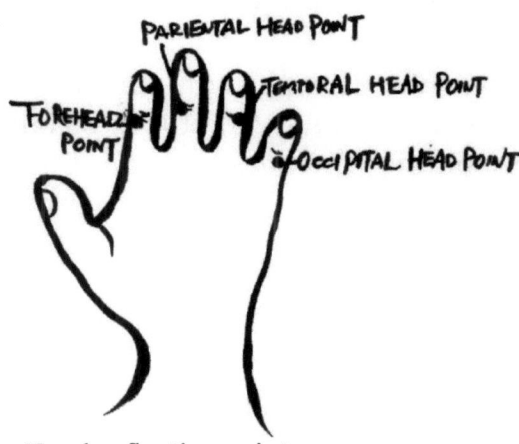

Head reflective point

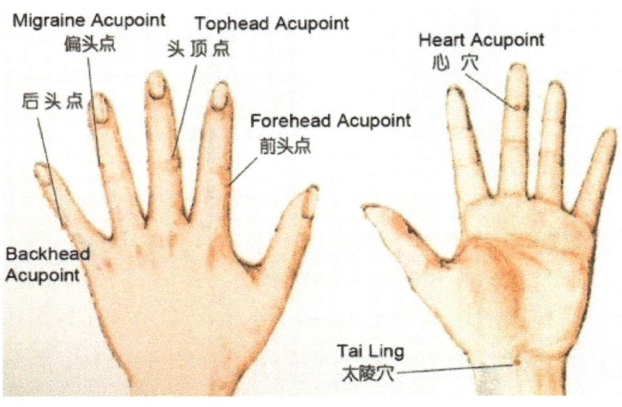

1-15 Insomnia 不寐 Bumei

In mild Insomnia, the patient may have difficulty falling asleep, and finds it difficult to go back to sleep. In severe Insomnia, the patient cannot fall asleep all night.

- Treatment
  Acupuncture point:
  P-6 (Neiguan 内关), HT-7 (Shenmen 神门)

  Massage:
  HT-7 (Shenmen 神门), P-9 (Zhongchong 中冲)
  Reflective point:

Heart point

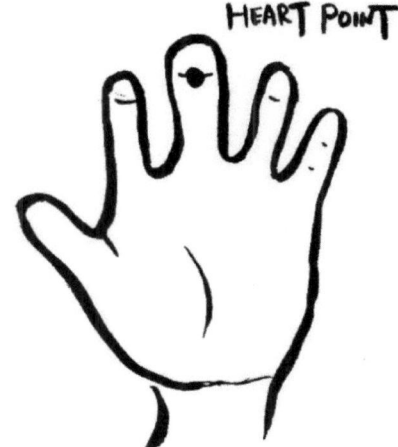

Heart reflective point

1-16 Lumbago 腰痛 **Yaotong**

The symptoms are pain in the waist area. This is the diseases of spinal column, injury of soft tissues beside spinal column, compression of spinal nerve roots or gynecological diseases.

- Treatment
  Acupuncture point:
  SI-6 (Yanglao 养老), SI-3 (Houxi 后溪)

Massage:
The strong stimulation is applied with Local massage
Reflective point:
Waist point

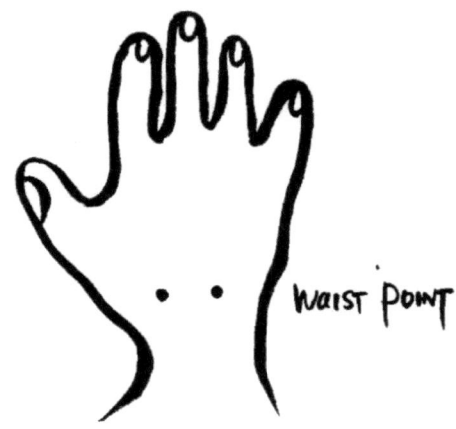

Waist reflective point

1-17 Retention of urine 癃闭 Longbi

This is with reduced discharge or complete cessation of urination.

- Treatment
  Acupuncture point:
  LU-11 (Shaoshang 少商), LI-4 (Hegu 合谷)

1-18 Stiff neck 落枕 Laozhen

It is caused by an increase of local muscular tension or static injury to local tissues after sleeping in an improper posture.

- Treatment
  Acupuncture point:
  SJ-5 (Waiguan 外关), SI-3 (Houxi 后溪), SJ-3 (Zhongdu 中诸)

  Reflective point:
  Neck point

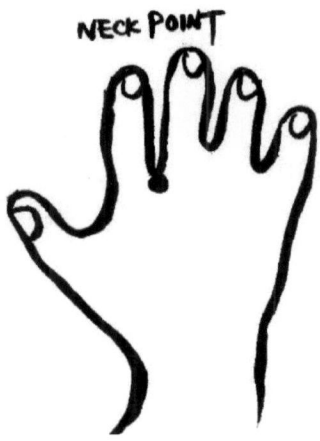

Neck reflective point

1-19 Psychosis 精神病 Jingshenbing

There is divided into two types.
1) It is characterized by an apathetic expression, silence, mental dullness, speaking nonsense, and diminished motion.

2) It is characterized by mental excitement, hyper-irritability, restlessness, noise making, beating and scolding others, destruction and extreme fury.

- Treatment
  Acupuncture point:
  LU-11 (Shaoshang 少商), HT-9 (Shaochong 少冲), P-9 (Zhongchong 中冲), SJ-1 (Guanchong 关冲)

  Reflective point:
  Heart point, Lung point, Spleen point, and liver point.

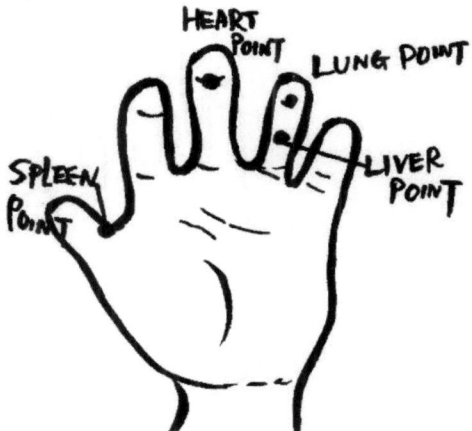

Heart, Spleen, Lung and Liver reflective point

1-20 Vomiting 呕吐 Outu

This is due to the adverse ascent of stomach Qi.

- Treatment
  Acupuncture point:
  P-6 (Neiguan 内关), P-7 (Daling 大陵)

  Massage:
  P-8 (Laogong 劳宫), P-7 (Daling 大陵), EX-UE-4
  (Zongkui 中魁), EX-UE 5 (Dagukong 大骨空)

  Reflective point:

Chest point

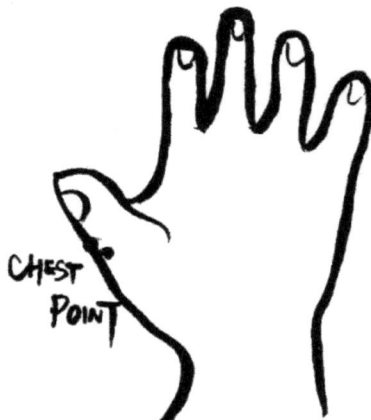

Chests point on palm and back of the hand reflective point

1-21 Shortness of breath 呼吸急促 Huxijicu

This is with repeated elevation of shoulders and flaring nostrils.

- Treatment
  Acupuncture point:
  LU-10 (Yuji 鱼际), LU-9 (Taiyuan 太渊)

  Massage: LU-11 (Shaoshang 少商), LU-9 (Taiyuan 太渊)
  Reflective point:

Lung point.

1-22 Heart palpitations 心悸 **Xinji**

This is with rapid heartbeat and sometimes loss of self-control, and often accompanied by insomnia, poor memory, and vertigo.

- Treatment
  Acupuncture point:
  P-6 (Neiguan 内关), HT-7 (Shenmen 神门)

  Massage:
  HT-7 (Shenmen 神门), HT-8 (Shaofu 少府)), P-7 (Daling 大陵), HT-9 (Shaochong 少冲)

  Reflective point:
  Heart point

1-23 Hiccups 呃逆 **Eni**

This is due to the adverse ascent of Qi from below. Hiccups occur in patients with neuroses of stomach and intestines, gastritis, gastric dilatation, liver cirrhosis at late stage, cerebrovascular disease, and uremia.

- Treatment
  Acupuncture point:
  P-6 (Neiguan 内关), EX-UE4 (Zhongkui 中魁),
  LI-4 (Hegu 合谷)

  Massage:
  P-8 (Laogong 劳宫), SI-2 (Qiangu 前谷), EX-UE4
  (Zhongkui 中魁)

  Reflective point:
  Hiccup point

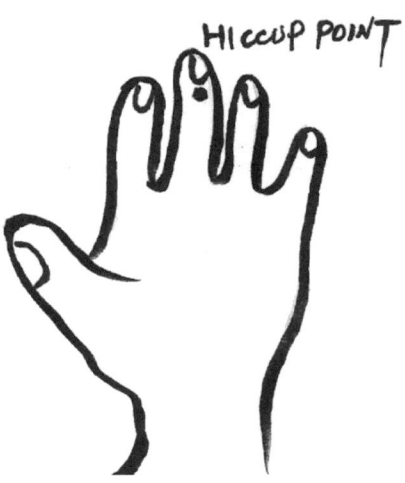

Hiccup reflective point

1-24 Cerebral apoplexy 脑卒中 Naocuzhong

It is also called stroke with symptoms of collapse, loss of consciousness, deviation of mouth and eye, hemiplegia and aphasia.

- Treatment
  Acupuncture point:
  (1) Internal organs: 12 Jing points, EX-UE11 (Shixuan 十宣)

  (2) Speech disturbance: HT 5 (Tongli 通里), P-6 (Neiguan 内关), LI-4 (Hegu 合谷)
  (3) Numbness and paralysis of upper limbs: LI-11 (Quchi 曲池), SJ-5 (Waiguan 外关), LI-4 (Hegu 合谷)

  (4) Contralateral side: SI-3 (Houxi 后溪)

  Massage:
  HT-7 (Shenmen 神门), LU-11 (Shaoshang 少商), LI-2 (Erjian 二间), LI-4 (Hegu 合谷), SI-1 (Shaoze 少泽), SI-2 (Qiangu 前谷)

1-25 Muscular atrophy 肌肉萎缩 **Jirou weisuo**

This is with flaccidity and weakness of muscles, and complete muscular atrophy.

- Treatment
  Acupuncture point:
  LI-11 (Quchi 曲池), SJ-5 (Waiguan 外关), LI-10 (Shousanli 手三里), LI-4 (Hegu 合谷)

1-26 Dementia 痴呆 **Chidai**

This is a neurological disease with mental dullness, silence, no desire to speak, and poor memory. Severe patients cannot take care of their daily needs and are in danger of injuring themselves.

- Treatment
  Acupuncture point:
  P-6 (Neiguan 内关), HT-7 (Shenmen 神门), LI-4 (Hegu 合谷)

  Reflective point:
  Heart and kidney point.

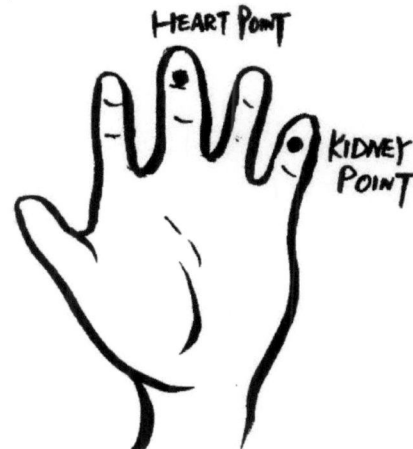

Heart and Kidney reflective point

1-27 Numbness 麻木 Mamu

This is loss of sensation in skin, muscles, and limbs. This causes that skin and muscles are in various diseases of connective tissue, nutritional, metabolic, and endocranial diseases.

- Treatment
  Acupuncture point:
  Upper limbs:

LI-11 (Quchi 曲池), LI-4 (Hegu 合谷), SJ-5 (Waiguan 外关)

Hands:
EX-UE-9 (Baxie 八邪), SI-3 (Houxi 后溪), P-6 (Neiguan 内关), LI-4 (Hegu 合谷),

Fingers:
EX-UE-11 (Shixuan 十宣)

Reflective area:
Areas corresponding to the region of numbness in dorsal reflective areas and radial or ulnar reverse dorsal reflective areas.

1-28 Febrile diseases 温病 Wenbing

This chronic diseases with fever caused by dysfunction of the internal organs and deficiency of Qi, blood, Yin and Yang. This includes low fever, tumors, hematological diseases, tuberculosis, endocranial diseases.

- Treatment
  Acupuncture point:

LI-11 (Quchi 曲池), LI-4 (Hegu 合谷), P-8 (Laogong 劳宫), LU-10 (Yuji 鱼际)

1-29 Malaria 疟疾 Nûeji

This is with chills, high fever, headache and profuse sweating.

- Treatment
  Acupuncture point:
  SI-3 (Houxi 后溪), P-5 (Jianshi 间使), LI-11 (Quchi 曲池)

1-30 Heat stroke 中暑 Zhongshu

This is a sudden onset of high fever, profuse sweating, mental confusion, sleepiness, and sometimes convulsions due to the attack of summer-heat pathogen.

- Treatment
  Acupuncture point:

EX-UE11 (Shixuan 十宣), LI-11 (Quchi 曲池), LI-4 (Hegu 合谷)

1-31 Costal pain 肋骨痛 Leigutong

Costal pain is closely related to the Liver and Gallbladder which meridians pass through the costal region. The Liver lies in the costal region with the Gallbladder attached to Liver.

- Treatment
  Acupuncture point:
  SJ-5 (Waiguan 外关), SJ-3 (Zhongdu 中诸), SJ-6 (Zhigou 支沟), SI-4 (Wangu 腕骨)

  Reflective point:
  Temporal head point.

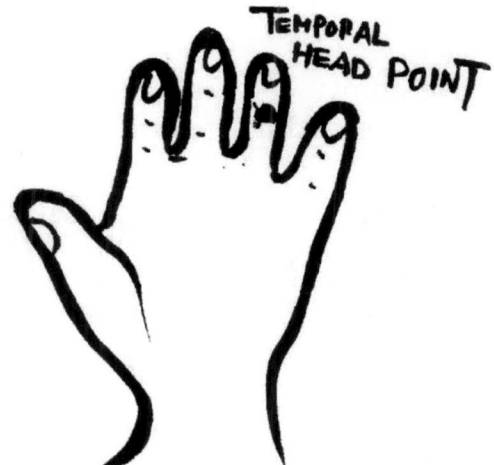

Temporal head reflective point

II. Gynecology
2-1 Amenorrhea 闭经 Bijing

This is a condition that menstruation has not begun in girls over 18 years, or menstruation stopped over three months.

- Treatment
  Acupuncture point:
  LI-4 (Hegu 合谷), SI-3 (Houxi 后溪)

Massage:
SI-3 (Houxi 后溪)

Reflective point:
Kidney, spine and liver point.

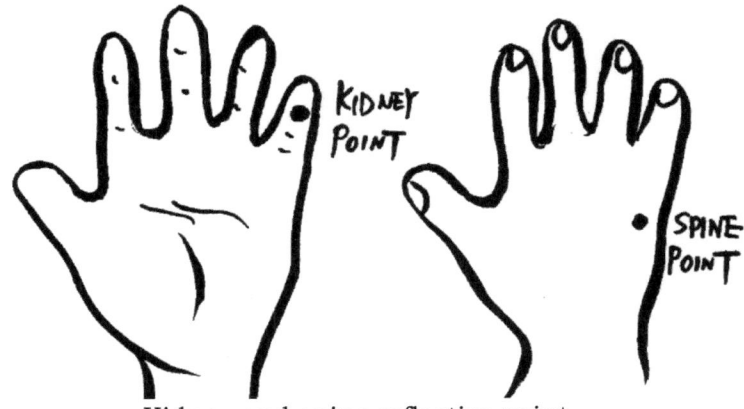

Kidney and spine reflective point

2-2 Dysmenorrhea 痛经 Tongjing

This is characterized by lower abdominal pain before, during, or after the menstrual period. The pain may radiate to lumbar and sacral regions, and severe pain may cause fainting.

- Treatment
  Acupuncture point:

LI-4 (Hegu 合谷)

Reflective point:
Sanjiao and waist point.

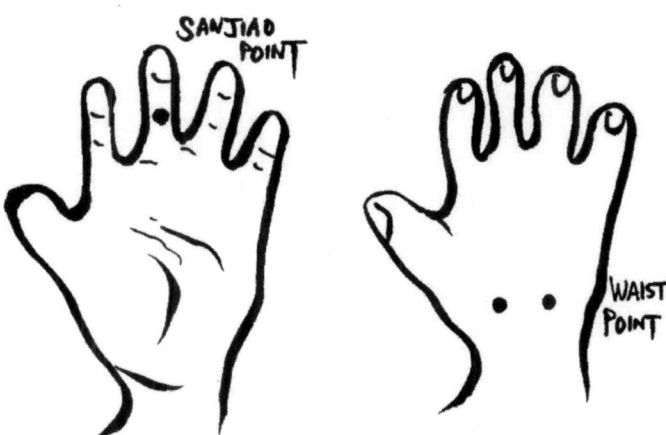

Sanjiao and waist reflective point

2-3 Postpartum 产后 Chanhou

After delivery, the mother may suddenly develop dizziness, blurred vision, chest distress, nausea, vomiting, shortness of breath with accumulation of phlegm, restlessness, or trismus, loss consciousness.

- Treatment
  Acupuncture point:

P-6 (Neiguan 内关), LI-4 (Hegu 合谷), LU-6 (Kongzui 孔最), HT-6 (Yinxi 阴郄)

Reflective point:
Heart, spleen, and kidney point.

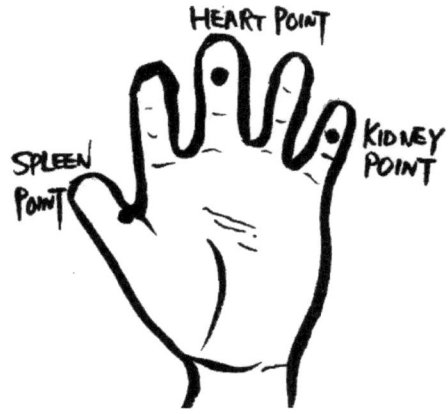

Heart, spleen, and kidney reflective point

2-4 Postpartum convulsions 产后抽出 Chanhou Chouchu

This is a condition with convulsions of the limbs, stiffness of neck and back.

- Treatment

Acupuncture point:
LI-11 (Quchi 曲池), LI-4 (Hegu 合谷), SI-3 (Houxi 后溪), P-6 (Neiguan 内关)

2-5 Menstrual headache 经期头痛 Jinqitoutong

This is a condition with headache before, during, or after the menstrual period due to blood deficiency, stagnant blood.

- Treatment
  Acupuncture point:
  LI-4 (Hegu 合谷), SI-3 (Houxi 后溪)

  Massage:
  LI-4 (Hegu 合谷), SI-1 (Shaoze 少泽), SI-2 (Qiangu 前谷), SI-3 (Houxi 后溪), SJ-2 (Yemen 液门)

  Reflective area:
  Head area corresponding to the location of headache in dorsal and palmar reflective areas.

III. Surgical and Dermatological Disease

3-1 Eczema 湿疹 Shizhen

This is a chronic, recurring and irritating skin disease.

- Treatment
  Acupuncture point:
  LI-11 (Quchi 曲池), LI-4 (Hegu 合谷), EX-UE1 (Zhoujian 肘尖)

  Massage:
  Tender spots, kidney, stomach, intestine, spleen, and lung area.

3-2 Herpes zoster 带状疱疹 Daizhuangpaozhen

This is an acute skin disease with burning pain. The skin lesions are the erythema and clusters of vesicles arranged in tapelike around the trunk of the body.

- Treatment
  LI-11 (Quchi 曲池)), LI-4 (Hegu 合谷), SJ-6
  (Zhigou 支沟), SJ-5 (Waiguan 外关), SI-3 (Houxi
  后溪)

  Reflective area:
  Areas corresponding to the location of lesion
  in dorsal and palmar reflective areas.

3-3 Urticaria 荨麻疹 Xunmazhen

This is a skin disease with pink or pale papules
appearing on the skin and then disappearing from
time to time.

- Treatment
  Acupuncture point:
  LI-11 (Quchi 曲池), LI-4 (Hegu 合谷), SI-3
  (Houxi 后溪)

  Massage:
  Lung, liver, stomach, intestine areas, and lung
  reflective point.

IV. Pediatric Diseases

4-1 Convulsions 小儿惊风 Xiaoerjingfeng

This is a common symptom in children with convulsions and mental confusion.

- Treatment
  Acupuncture point:
  Twelve Jing-Well* points, EX-UE-11 (Shixuan 十宣), P-6 (Neiguan 内关), LI-4 (Hegu 合谷)

  *12 Jing-Well points:
  LU-11 (Shaoshang 少商), SP-1 (Yinbai 隐白), HT-9 (Shaochong 少冲), KI-1 (Yongquan 涌泉), P-9 (Zhongchong 中冲), LIV-1 (Dadun 大敦), LI-1 (Shangyang 商阳), ST-45 (Lidui 历兑), SI-1, (Shaoze 少泽), BL-67 (Zhiyin 至阴), SJ-1 (Guanchong 关冲), GB-44 (Zuqiaoyin 足窍阴)
  The needles are inserted for 1.6 cm and retained for five minutes after twisting, lifting, and thrusting stimulation.

4-2 Anorexia 厌食症 Yashizheng

This is characterized by poor appetite and refusal to eat over a long period of time.

- Treatment
  Acupuncture point:
  LI-10 (Shousanli 手三里), LI-4 (Hegu 合谷), EX-UE10 (Sifeng 四缝)
  The needles are shallowly inserted, but not retained.

  Reflective points:
  Stomach and intestine, and spleen points.

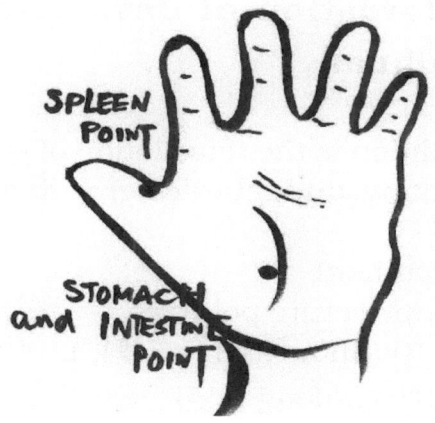

Stomach and Intestine, and spleen point

4-3 Infantile malnutrition 小儿营养不良 Yingyangbuliang

This is a common for children with general weakness and pathological leanness, sallow complexion, and dry hair due to improper feeding.

- Treatment
  Acupuncture point:
  EX-UE10 (Sifeng 四缝)
  The needles are shallowly inserted, but not retained.

4-4 Retardation of development 发育迟缓 Fayuchihuan

This condition is the retardation of standing, walking, and speaking, and retarded growth of hair and teeth.

- Treatment
  Acupuncture point:
  LI-10 (Shousanli 手三里), LI-4 (Hegu 合谷), EX-UE-10 (Sifeng 四缝)

The needles are shallowly inserted, but not retained.

4-5 Stagnation of food 食物停滞 Shiwutingzhi

The symptoms are poor appetite, indigestion, abdominal distension, and irregular bowel movement.

- Treatment
  Acupuncture point:
  EX-UE 10, LI-4 (Hegu 合谷)
  The needles of LI-4 (Hegu 合谷) are shallowly inserted, but not retained

4-6 Weakness 虚弱 Xuruo

This includes with weakness of neck, mouth, arms, legs and muscles.

- Treatment
  Acupuncture point:

LI-11 (Quchi 曲池), P-6 (Neiguan 内关), SI-3 (Houxi 后溪), LI-4 (Hegu 合谷)

Moxibution can be applied at above acupoints.

V. Diseases of the Eye, Ear, Nose, Throat and Oral Cavity

5-1 Glaucoma 青光眼 Qingguangyan

This is an eye with tense eyeball, dilated and greenish pupil, and marked impairment of vision. It is often caused by emotional excitement or over fatigue, and in the early stages the patient may suffer from slight distension of eyeball, ipsilateral frontal headache, soreness of the nose, and blurred vision.

- Treatment
  Acupuncture point:
  LI-4 (Hegu 合谷)
  Massage:
  EX-UE5 (Dagukong 大骨空), EX-UE6 (Xiaogukong 小骨空), LI-1 (Shangyang 商阳), SI-1 (Shaoze 少泽), SI-3 (Houxi 后溪)

Reflective points:
Eye and liver points.

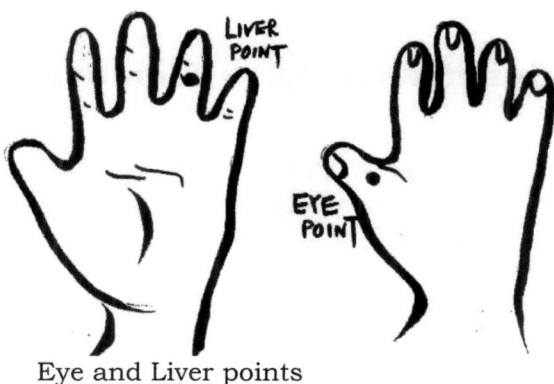

Eye and Liver points

5-2 Myopia 近视 Jinshi

This is a condition with normal near sight but impaired far sight.

- Treatment
  Acupuncture point:
  LI-4 (Hegu 合谷)
  Massage
  LI-2 (Erjian 二间), EX-UE5 (Dagukong 大骨空),
  EX-UE6 (Xiaogukong 小骨空)

Reflective points:
Eye area in palmar reflective areas and ulnar or radial reverse palmar reflective areas.

5-3 Conjunctivitis 结膜炎 Jiemoyan

This is an acute eye with redness, swelling, hotness, and pain in the eyes caused by external wind and heat pathogens.

- Treatment
  Acupuncture point:
  SJ-1 (Guanchong 关冲), LI-1 (Shangyang 商阳), LI-4 (Hegu 合谷)

  Reflective points:
  Eye and liver points.

5-4 Strabismus 斜视 Xieshi

This is sudden onset of eyeball deviation with limited eyeball movement and double vision.

- Treatment
  Acupuncture point:

SJ-3 (Zhongdu 中诸), LI-4 (Hegu 合谷)

Reflective points:
Eye and liver points.

5-5 Sore throat 咽喉肿 Yanhouzhongtong

This is the throat with redness, swelling and pain.

- Treatment
  Acupuncture point:
  LI-4 (Hegu 合谷), LU-11 (Shaoshang 少商), LI-1 (Shangyang 商阳)

5-6 Tinnitus and deafness 耳鸣 耳聋 Erming Erlong

- Treatment
  Acupuncture point:
  SJ-2 (Yemen 液门), SJ-3 (Zhongdu 中诸), SJ-5 (Waiguan 外关)
  Massage:
  LI-1 (Shangyang 商阳), LI-4 (Hegu 合谷), LI-5 (Yangxi 阳溪), SI-2 (Qiangu 前谷), SI-3 (Houxi

后溪), SI-4 (Wangu 腕骨), SI-5 (Yanggu 阳谷), SJ-3 (Zhongdu 中诸), SJ-4 (Yangchi 阳池)
Reflective points:
Temporal head and kidney points.

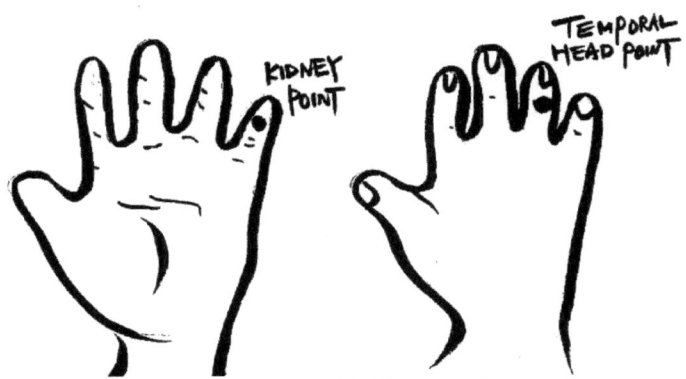

Temporal head and kidney points

5-7 Laryngitis 喉炎 Houyan

This is an acute condition with hoarse voice and dysphonia.

- Treatment
  Acupuncture point:
  P-6 (Neiguan 内关), LI-4 (Hegu 合谷), LI-1 (Shangyang 商阳), LU-11 (Shaoshang 少商)

Reflective points:
Throat and tonsil points.

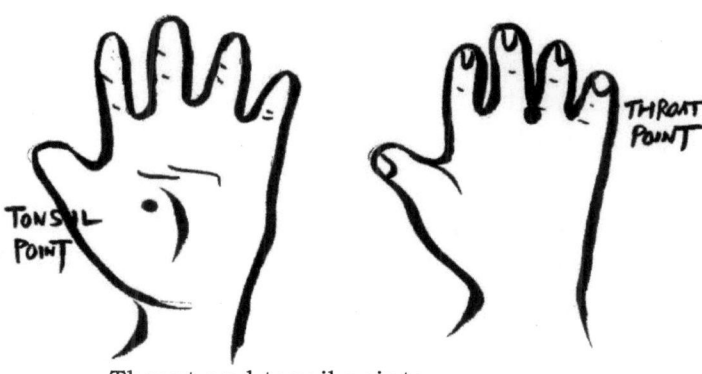

Throat and tonsil points

5-8 Deviation of mouth (Facial palsy) 面瘫 Miantan

This is with deviation of mouth and eye.

- Treatment
  Acupuncture point:
  LI-4 (Hegu 合谷), LI-11 (Quchi 曲池)
  Massage:
  LI-2 (Erjian 二间), LI-4 (Hegu 合谷)
  Reflective areas:
  The corresponding areas of the face in the palmar reflective areas and ulnar or radial reverse palmar reflective areas.

5-9 Toothache 牙痛 Yatong

This is a symptom of various diseases of the teeth and periodontal structures.

- Treatment
  Acupuncture point:
  LI-1 (Shangyang 商阳), LI-4 (Hegu 合谷)
  Massage:
  LI-1 (Shangyang 商阳), LI-4 (Hegu 合谷), LI-2 (Erjian 二间), LI-3 (Sanjian 三间), LI-5 (Yangxi 阳溪) SI-3 (Houxi 后溪)

  Reflective point:
  Toothache point.

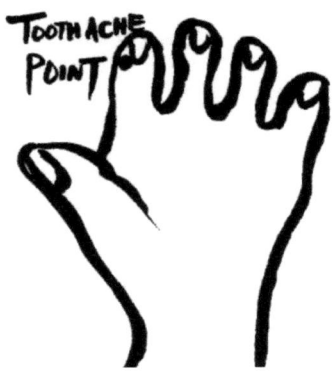

References 参考文献

1. Zhou Qinghui, Wrist-Ankle Acupuncture, 2002.

2. Wang Sheng, Hand Therapy, 1997.

3. Musculoskeletal Key.

4. E. Akimoto, Hand and Foot point.

5. Hand reflective zones chart.

Other library of Traditional Chinese Medicine by Sumiko Knudsen

1. Acupuncture for Weight Loss
2. Akupunkture til Vægttab
3. Acupuncture Meridians and Points
4. Akupunktur Meridianer og Punkter
5. Ear Acupuncture
6. Øre Akupunktur
7. Body Acupuncture, Clinical Treatment
8. Krop Akupunktur, Klinisk Behandling
9. Acupuncture and Moxibustion
10. Akupunktur og Moxibustion
11. Scalp Acupuncture
12. Hovedbundsakupunktur